FOLK MEDICINE

A Vermont Doctor's Guide to Good Health

FOLK MEDICINE

A Vermont Doctor's Guide

to Good Health

By D. C. JARVIS, M.D.

HOLT, RINEHART AND WINSTON

NEW YORK / CHICAGO / SAN FRANCISCO

Library of Congress Catalog Card Number: 58-6454

Published, February, 1958

ISBN: 0-03-027410-9

Printed in the United States of America

This book is dedicated to
my daughter, Sylvia Jarvis Smith, and my grandson,
Jarvis Fred Smith
To convey to them through the written word
the folk medicine of Vermont
which one generation of native Vermonters, living close
to the soil, hands on by word of mouth to
succeeding generations.

Foreword

I AM A FIFTH-GENERATION Vermonter on my mother's side. My medical-college and internship days in Burlington trained me in organized medicine. When I located in Barre, to pursue my chosen specialty of eye, ear, nose and throat, I recognized another type of medicine which I had to know and understand if I was to gain the medical confidence and respect of my fellow Vermonters who lived close to the soil on back-road farms. This medicine—Vermont folk medicine—had not been part of my formal training, but it is deeply a part of Vermont living. I set about learning it and understanding its origins.

My studies led me to considerable readjustment of orthodox approaches. For example, it did not immediately make medical sense to me that a sore throat could be cured in one day by chewing fresh gum of the spruce tree. But I saw that I would be wise to learn the principles of this folk medicine and cultivate a willingness to prescribe its time-honored remedies where precedent indicated that they would be as, or more, efficacious than the remedies which organized medicine had taught me to use.

When I discussed a variety of specific treatments of this indigenous medicine with my colleagues at regional and national medical-society meetings, they asked me to continue the discussion at greater length by starting a correspondence study group, basing letters on my cumulative findings. I carried on this correspondence for twenty years. Membership was limited to fifty persons. Practically all were nationally known; many were faculty members of medical schools. The letters went out Tuesdays and Fridays to a mailing list in thirty-two states.

I conceived this book originally to pass on to my daughter and her descendents the principles and workings of this folk medicine as tested in the course of my practice. Later I decided to expand it. My wish for it is that it may bring knowledge and understanding of the nature and long-successful uses of folk medicine to anyone interested in daily increased vitality from childhood through maturity to satisfyingly active old age.

I believe that the doctor of the future will be a teacher as well as physician. His real job will be to teach people how to be healthy. Doctors will be even busier than they are now because it is a lot harder to keep people well than it is to just get them over a sickness.

Vermont folk medicine has much to give those who reject as inevitable the specter of physical impairment and weakening, and who prefer instead to plan to be strong, active, and free from disease to the very end of their days.

D. C. JARVIS

Barre, Vermont
December 5, 1957

Contents

FOLK MEDICINE

A Vermont Doctor's Guide to Good Health

CHAPTER I

Definitions

FOLK MEDICINE REACHES very far back in time. Nature opened the first drugstore. Primitive man and the animals depended on preventive use of its stock of plants and herbs to avoid disease and to maintain health and vigor. Because man and the animals were constantly on the move, Nature's drugstore had branches everywhere. Wherever in the world you were sick, you would find in the fields its medicines to cure you, its materials for curative herbal teas and ointments.

Vermont folk medicine has been unfolding in the *Ver-* (green) *mont* (mountains) since aboriginal times. It adapts very old physiological and biochemical laws to the maintenance of health and vigor in the environmental conditions of Vermont living. But there is no geographical limit on the laws, and their applications will work well in many environments.

As with all folk medicine from time immemorial, the ideal of Vermont folk medicine is to condition the body in its entirety so that disease will not attack it. Now and then one finds people taking it for granted that "folk medicine" is a vague term for a collection of medical old wives' tales. It is inevitable that some myths would creep in along the way. For example, when I was a child, a string of Job's Tears— a species of grass having round, shiny grains imaginatively said to resemble the patient tears of the sorely tried Old

Testament character—frequently were hung by a mother around the neck of her child "to help him cut his teeth." And of course all of us have heard of the supposedly magical, if smelly, powers of a little sack of asafoetida—the gum-resin substance with the garlicky odor—which, worn around the neck through the cold winter months, would surely repel sickness. In considering folk medicine, obviously witch-doctor myths should be separated from the genuine article.

Our pioneer ancestors discovered the rudiments of their folk medicine in the healing plants sought out by animals suffering from alimentary disturbances, fever, and wounds. By observing how animals cure themselves from disease, they learned how to keep themselves healthy by Nature's own methods.

I have come to marvel at the instinct of animals to make use of natural laws for healing themselves. They know unerringly which herbs will cure what ills. Wild creatures first seek solitude and absolute relaxation, then they rely on the complete remedies of Nature—the medicine in plants and pure air. A bear grubbing for fern roots; a wild turkey compelling her babies in a rainy spell to eat leaves of the spice bush; an animal, bitten by a poisonous snake, confidently chewing snakeroot—all these are typical examples. An animal with fever quickly hunts up an airy, shady place near water, there remaining quiet, eating nothing but drinking often until its health is recovered. On the other hand, an animal bedeviled by rheumatism finds a spot of hot sunlight and lies in it until the misery bakes out.

In Vermont, accepting Nature's well-worked-out plan for good health and freedom from disease as observed in animals, people simply follow the plan, not trying continually to revise it in accordance with some whim of their own. Thus they carry over into adult life instincts and habits from their childhood.

The body needs assistance to meet the complications, stresses and strains of modern civilization. Mercifully during childhood we are more or less protected by instincts. But when we leave the world of childhood, we are all too prone to consider these instincts old-fashioned. Happily it is never too late to relearn them, if we are willing to observe the way Nature's laws are followed by animals and by little children.

If you care to go to school to the bees, the fowl, the cats, dogs, goats, mink, calves, dairy cows, bulls, and horses, and allow them to teach you their ways, as have generations of Vermonters living by the prescriptions of Vermont folk medicine, you will gain insight into a physiological and biochemical medicine not to be learned from medical books. Verified through observing results in animals, this medicine, which has passed from generation to generation by word of mouth, enables great numbers of Vermonters to continue carrying heavy daily work loads and to go on well past the Scriptural three-score-and-ten years with good physical and mental vigor, good digestion, good eyesight, and good hear-ing, avoiding senility to the very end.

Having defined the broad nature of folk medicine and specified the Vermont version of it, this book proposes to discuss it in a light which will enable any reader to better understand problems of the body in relation to living. This is done with the hope that rough places in your life pathway may be made smoother, and you may come into the latter years with a still-efficient human machine, represented by your body.

CHAPTER II

Vermont Environment and the Life Span

VERMONT FOLK MEDICINE has evolved out of a blend of Nature's preventive and curative principles, common sense, and the hard fact that Vermont is climatically one of the most unstable areas in the world.

In our latitude the prevailing winds are westerly. Of the twenty-six storm tracks crossing the United States on their way to the Atlantic Ocean, twenty-three pass over Vermont. Consequently Vermont weather changes every few days the year round, and the Vermonter faces the major biological necessity of constantly adjusting his body to rapidly alternating heat and cold, high and low barometric pressure, and seasonal changes of humidity and air ionization. Every such adjustment to climate must be made by a change in the blood circulation. One day the skin is called upon to be a radiator, giving off heat. The next day it may have to be an insulator, retaining the body heat. This puts great strain on the heart and blood vessels.

According to American Heart Association statistics, Vermont has a good deal of heart disease directly attributable to climatic instability. Vermont folk medicine includes ways to aid the heart, the blood vessels, and the blood supply, so

6

that heart attacks may be avoided, the heart will not wear out as quickly, and its life may be prolonged.

Your heart is the motor of your human machine. The body muscles, including that muscle which is the heart, work on sugar. The researchers of our folk medicine, noting effects of environment, food, and variations in food on animals and humans, show that it makes a great difference to your heart whether you give it the natural sugar which is found in honey, or refined white sugar. You can be kind to your heart by giving it honey on which to do its work.

When working normally your heart is capable of pumping six ounces of blood per heartbeat into the large artery leaving the heart. The amount of sugar in your blood is one teaspoonful. This amount is so essential that, were it reduced to a half teaspoonful, you would lose consciousness. If it were increased for any length of time to more than one teaspoonful, diabetes might make its appearance. Clearly you need to give careful thought to what you give your body, to make sure this teapsoonful of sugar is constantly in your blood.

Nature intended not only that we have sugar for immediate use by the heart but that we also have a thin trickle of sugar going through the intestinal wall all the time. In honey we have two sugars, one called *dextrose,* the other called *levulose.* Dextrose constitutes 40 per cent of honey, levulose 34 per cent. When honey is taken, dextrose passes swiftly into the blood. Levulose, being more slowly absorbed, maintains a steady level of blood sugar concentration. It keeps honey from raising the blood sugar level farther than can be dealt with by the body.

Vermont is second among the states of the nation in percentage of population over the age of sixty-five. Not long ago it had 40,000 persons over that age, and each year nearly 2500 reach it.

Eighteen per cent of Vermont's population is over fifty-

five years of age. One survey of ministers in the Vermont
Methodist Church Conference showed, for a ten-year period,
that the average age at death of Methodist ministers was
eighty years, and that several in this group lived beyond the
age of ninety.

Men in their seventies do a full day's work on Vermont
farms as a matter of course, and it is not unusual to find men
of eighty sharing the farm work as though they were many
years younger. These Vermonters are helped to prolong their
working years by applying physiological and biochemical
laws they see at work in Nature.

It is accepted in Vermont as the rule that an animal's minimum life is five times the period required for it to mature.
A chicken, mature at six months, easily lives to an age of two
and one-half years. A dog, mature at one year, easily lives to
be five years old. A calf, mature at two years and going into
production at two and one-half years, lives to be twelve; and
a horse, mature at four years, will live to be twenty. Many
live longer.

Turning to the human animal, what do we find?

We note that the first twenty years of life are devoted to
the development of heart and blood-vessel capacity, digestive
and eliminative efficiency, mental and physical capacity, and
the emotions of self-perpetuation and self-defense.

In terms of the norm with animals, the rule for the human
life span, being five times twenty, would be one hundred
years.

What happens after the twenty-year mark?

Often we find that while a man's mental vigor and life
purpose continue to expand, the physical equipment begins
to deteriorate. Therefore an upward line, representing
mental vigor and life purpose, and a downward line, representing deterioration of physical equipment, cross at the
age of fifty years. By the age of sixty he often finds himself in
a semi-invalid condition, unable to do his best work.

Vermonters learn to prolong the working years. Instead

of crossing at the age of fifty, the upward and downward line will not cross before the age of eighty. A man may do his best work in the period from sixty to eighty years because his mental vigor and purpose remain at their best while he has maintained the physical equipment enabling him to carry on his business or profession, or, if he retires, to enjoy his retirement. The folk medicine practiced in Vermont aims at a goal of living wherein a man may live five times the period of time required for him to mature, as do the animals.

That it is possible to prolong the span of life beyond seventy years of age is amply proved by studying native Vermonters living close to the soil. The more I have studied, the more I have observed the close relation between prolongation of the life span and the daily intake of food. The Vermonter's knowledge of food has not come out of books but from close association with the creatures of the barnyard, which teaches that the daily food intake must be high in carbohydrates, represented by fruits, berries, edible leaves, and roots, and low in proteins, represented by meat, fowl, and eggs.

Vermonters accept the body tissues as soil in human form. Management of the soil to its best advantage requires understanding of natural laws, and specific care to maintain and rebuild it. On occasion you will hear a Vermonter speak of "my human house."

Common sense based on Nature's wise principles enables us to maintain and rebuild the human house for prolonged habitation. Its efficiency and duration depend on the wise selection of foods eaten, liquids taken, and air breathed.

When you go about constructing a wooden building to dwell in, do you order just wood, any wood? Of course not. You begin with the understanding that different woods will be needed in the various parts of the building to meet the different problems of stress and strain. In Vermont we order pine floors, chestnut for woodwork, hemlock for joists, cedar for shingles.

To build and rebuild our human house, maintaining its efficiency and prolonging our title to occupancy, we take into account dominance of the body by mineral elements. These minerals, steadily present in the body, keep it functioning smoothly. We speak of it as "making living worthwhile." The number of minerals included in the functioning of the human body is one of the wonders of life. Except for silver and gold, practically all minerals are in action.

In Vermont folk medicine there is an extremely simple prescription for replenishing the mineral needs of the body. It is as follows: two teaspoonfuls of honey and two teaspoonfuls of apple cider vinegar, taken in a glass of water one or more times each day, depending on how much mental and physical work is done. The blend tastes like a glass of apple cider. The vinegar brings across from the apple its mineral content, the honey brings across the minerals in the nectar of flowers.

CHAPTER III

The Animal Laws

MAN TENDS TO BE a rebel against Nature and a deserter from the animal kingdom. In the light of this fact let us consider the animal laws, which apply to man as well as to animals. Farm animals are a good example of these laws. In their own way cattle, horses, hogs, and other domestic livestock are just as natural as the wild animals which roam the untouched forests; and if we will but take the trouble to study them, they can teach us many valuable lessons. Country children know this. City children, having missed the close touch of daily association with farm animals, often grow up without any knowledge of the animal laws.

Take an animal's refusal to eat when it is sick. By letting food alone, it creates within its body a new biochemical state which assists in hastening recovery. When we are sick, fearing to seem lacking in appreciation, we often will eat food brought to us. Thus we are acting in direct opposition to the animal laws. If we wish to imitate the animals' restorative biochemical change within the body, we can do so by limiting ourselves to an acid drink such as grape juice, which contains tartaric acid; or cranberry juice, which contains citric, malic, quinic and benzoic acids; or to apple juice, which contains malic acid.

Humans have a habit of feeling that if they omit a meal something terrible will happen to them. They do not remember that the body stores reserves against time of need

11

and could maintain itself, if necessary without taking any food whatever, for the length of time of the average sickness. They fail to realize that through the first twenty years of life more food may be required as building material. By the time they have reached the age of twenty-five the bony framework, muscle system, heart and blood-vessel system, and respiratory and digestive systems are built. What is needed from that point is a daily food selection representing maintenance of the different systems.

By the age of fifty one needs to begin building the body anew, not eating to gratify the appetite, but rather selecting the foods which our somber second thoughts tell us represent the elementary composition of the human body. By taking thought we can rebuild the body as we would rebuild a house.

Let us consider, too, the question of sleeping with the window open, summer and winter. In the past we have been taught that it would aid in preserving health to sleep with the window open the year round.

Years ago, after attending a course given by the Trudeau School of Tuberculosis at Saranac Lake, New York, I was impressed with the idea of advising my patients to sleep with the window open at night to aid continued good health. Subsequently I examined 500 granite cutters for the National Tuberculosis Association's Committee on Tuberculosis in the Dusty Trades. This group represented fourteen nationalities. Many of the men had emigrated to the United States, bringing with them customs of their native countries. A four-page examination form had to be filled out for each man examined, and one of the questions to be answered was, "Do you sleep with the window open at night?" The next question was, "Do you have frequent head colds?" After examining one hundred of the men I noted that those who slept with the window open at night had frequent head colds, and those who slept with the window closed did not. When the examination of the 500 men had been completed, we reached the conclusion that a relationship existed between sleeping with open windows and frequent head colds.

At about this time I was given the medical care of students in a private college-preparatory school. The headmaster wished me to study the common cold, which accounted for a great deal of time lost from classes. Among other measures a campaign was started for the open window at night, to help prevent head colds. Windows were open at night in all rooms but one. This room was occupied by two boys from farms. When they refused to sleep with the window open, I asked their reason. It was one I had never heard. "Doctor," they said, "we're trying to imitate the hen when we sleep at night. Do you know why she sleeps with her beak tucked in her feathers? We think she knows what she's doing. We'd like to know your idea of her reason."

I have lived long enough to be no stranger to youth's passion for having a bit of fun with the older generation. But they had certainly caught me unprepared. "Well," I said, "you've given me something to think about, all right. As soon as I find an answer I'll let you know." I lost no time in going to the animals to observe their sleeping habits.

The only answer that seems reasonable is that the hen tucks her beak into her feathers so that when she sleeps she will breathe warm fresh air. The air is drawn off the surface of her feathers and warmed as she exhales. It does not cool off before she inhales, with the result that her air supply is evenly warm, not cold.

Farmers tell me that the fox instinctively governs its air supply for sleeping in the same way. A fox, sleeping on top of the ground, will cover its face with its bushy tail so that the air it breathes will be fresh but warm. We have seen horses in an open field on a cold day. They stand with their heads close together. As they breathe out, the air circulating about their heads will not cool off very much before they breathe in again. A horse stands with its back to the wind on a cold, windy day.

Now there are, of course, people who thrive on sleeping with windows open to cold air straight through the coldest months of the year. They are like the fir tree on the mountainside, which endures harsh treatment and continues to flourish. They are the exception to the rule. But in the last analysis we are all subject to the animal laws.

Turning to the subject of exercise, we can study the animals too and note what they do. First of all, they roam the fields in search of food, which means they walk a great deal. A young animal is extremely active. Puppies and kittens are forever on the go, running, climbing, tussling, exploring. With the passing years body activity is directed toward securing food and defending itself and its offspring against enemy attack.

If we would take a leaf out of the animal book we would walk more. One ideal exercise would be gardening, for gardening uses the human body as roaming the fields for food uses the animal body.

We learn from studies of animals that the origin of leisure time was the resting of the body so that it might be in readiness to seek food or fight to defend itself. We learn also that the animal coat thickens with the approach of cold weather and thins when warmer months draw near. We too should vary the weight of our clothing with the changes of the seasons.

With the changing seasons, when their systems require certain adjustments, unerring instinct causes animals to change their diet. When they are on their own none of the foods they find are refined. They are not finicky, and they accept food in a natural state as Nature prepared it for them. For example, all female birds know by instinct that they need lime to form eggshells. It is common to see them resorting in mating season to places where shellfish will be found. Needing the lime, they follow Nature's guidebook to obtain it.

CHAPTER IV

Your Beginning

IT IS SOMETIMES DIFFICULT to grasp that once we were microscopic specks. Oliver Wendell Holmes used to say that the life of the individual begins a hundred years before he is born. It is certain that we do not start physiologically at birth, but nine months before coming into the world. The speck which is our beginning becomes alive through foods. It takes shelter, steady warmth, elimination of waste, and a healthy mother eating healthy foods to give an infant a good start.

If one hopes to be a successful gardener one soon learns in the garden the necessity of reinforcing soil with nitrogen, phosphorus and potassium. The nitrogen is for leaf growth; the phosphorus is to produce flowers; the potassium is for strength of root and stem. In proportion as any of these elements are left out, the plant will suffer.

Similarly, when one or more of the minerals needed by the infant in gestation are left out of the expectant mother's daily food intake, the building of the infant body will suffer.

Naturally the mother wishes a strong, vigorous baby at birth. She wishes an easy, short labor, and quick recovery of strength following it. This is a primitive inheritance. Tribal life was always on the move and there was no time to wait while women had long pregnancies and were slow in being able to get up and move on.

Today the daily intake of food is a large factor in an easy, short labor and quick recovery of strength. Wheat cereals and foods should be exchanged for rye or corn bread. Milk forms a curd in the stomach and should be exchanged for cheese, which does not. Muscle meats, such as beef, lamb and pork, should be exchanged for fish and other seafood, and such animal elements as liver, heart, kidneys and tripe. Honey should replace white sugar. Two raw vegetables and an egg should be taken daily. Vegetable salads supply leaves of plants containing vital minerals. The egg includes every element to form the chicken and is a complete food also for humans. Liver, once a week, is a "storehouse" food, but if one is unable to eat it the equivalent for daily intake can be found in one or two slices of liverwurst. Fowl should be eaten occasionally, nuts frequently. Citrus fruits, such as oranges and grapefruit, and citrus juices should be replaced with grape, apple, or cranberry juice, all prime sources of the minerals required by the developing infant.

Honey is not only an excellent food, it is a food supplement too. It prevents fermentation in the gastrointestinal tract and is quickly absorbed. Honey contains important elements for forming new blood. Having a mild laxative effect, it prevents constipation. Being also a body sedative, it helps to produce sound and refreshing sleep. And, returning to foods contributing to the pre-birth growth of the infant, two teaspoonfuls of honey, if taken at each meal either as a food sweetener or direct from the spoon, enable the developing infant to build a good nervous system.

When it comes to needed acids the expectant mother may figuratively be said to be in clover. Nature spreads acid about with a lavish hand in the foods that are the natural product of the soil. If there is a tendency to neglect the fruits, berries, and plant leaves that are a prime source of acids, the deficiency can be made up by a teaspoonful of apple cider vinegar to a glass of water, taken immediately on rising in the morning. Usually this mixture will incidentally prevent or clear up any morning sickness. During the day a glass of either cranberry, apple, or grape juice should be taken.

An expectant mother who makes a point of daily receiving the elements prescribed by Nature may expect to find the following when her infant is born:

It will have so much hair on its head that it will need a haircut the day it is born.

Fingernails will be strong, and long enough to need cutting.

The infant will have such a strong muscle system that it will be able to raise its head off the pillow of its own accord before it is a week old. As it grows a fine coordination between brain and muscles will be evident.

The mother should have plenty of milk, enabling her to nurse the baby if she wishes to do so.

The baby will digest and eliminate as a baby normally should.

The baby will have a good width of face.

Each jaw will be shaped like a horseshoe, as it should be, enabling each tooth to come through without crowding by other teeth.

Best of all, the child will be mentally bright. When its time comes to start school, it will be a pleasure to watch how well the child does.

The infant's teeth will reveal whether the mother's diet was or was not what it should have been. The teeth, formed while the infant is in the mother's body, are inside the gums at birth. When they come through they indicate whether the mother's blood carried correct food or not. When there is a good pre-natal foundation bad dietary conditions after birth do not easily upset it. There is no substitute for the perfect start, though in our modern civilization it is too often missed.

There are many common denominators in pregnancies of cows and of women. I owe to cows many of the observations which I apply to pregnant women and infants. I remember an example of short labor pointed out to me by a farmer after I recommended that he reinforce the cattle food with a daily ration of apple cider vinegar.

We happened to be chatting one day in his barn. He looked out into the lane and called my attention to a cow beginning to go into labor. He figured he had time to finish cleaning the stalls before going out to her. But in a few minutes, when he looked out into the lane again, the cow was on her feet, her calf beside her, walking toward the barn. The calf's coat was thick, the legs strong; all in all, an ideal working of Nature's plan.

In considering the human body we come to the realization that its health or sickness can be traced as far down as the minutest part of the body, the cell. Billions of microscopic organisms called *cells* make up the body. They are of various classes. There are muscle cells, nerve cells, bone cells, and the myriad cells which circulate throughout the body in the blood stream. Every single cell has its appointed share in the maintenance and well-being of the body as a whole.

Every body cell must live in a liquid medium. Because every cell is surrounded by fluid and the fluid is in constant motion, no two cells are ever in such close contact as to halt the flow. The manner in which fluid reaches the variously situated cells is unique. The arteries leave the heart to carry the blood to all the body tissues. Gradually they break up into smaller and smaller vessels until they become very fine, hairlike tubes called *capillaries.* These are so multitudinous that it would be practically impossible to pierce any body tissue with the finest needle without rupturing one or more of them.

Every cell selects out of the fluid the food and oxygen it needs to support its cell life, secreting back into the fluid all waste produced by its vital activity. The reason the fluid must constantly circulate is that, if it should stop, cells might languish and even die, not alone from stoppage of nutrition and oxygen but because they would be engulfed by poisonous waste materials.

Vermont folk medicine believes that disease begins when and because factors of the fundamental laws of life are interfered with. This is another way of holding that Vermont folk medicine places the burden for health or sickness on the nutrition of the body cells.

Disease does not come upon us unprovoked, like a thief in the night. Before harmful microorganisms can attack, multiply, thrive, and destroy, they must get into the cells. Our first thought when sickness appears, therefore, is to come to the rescue of the body cells. One way this can be done is by increasing intake of fluid which is acid in reaction, such as apple juice, cranberry, or grape juice; for Vermont folk medicine knows that acid thins the body fluids, keeping them liquid, while alkaline fluids thicken them, impeding circulation. Other ways are to increase the bowel action with a cathartic, and the skin action by sweating.

The application of Nature's laws for providing congenial conditions for growth are endless. I have selected several examples.

When I began the study of a mixed herd of 54 dairy cows the owner told me that 23 of them would not start a new pregnancy. Some of them had failed to do so for as long a period as one year. These cows had turned into mere boarders, and it was upsetting his herd milk-production program. He requested my help.

I suggested that for each twice-daily feeding he pour two ounces of apple cider vinegar over the ration of each of the 23 cows, immediately after the ration was placed in the feed trough. I also suggested that the herd bull have two ounces of apple cider vinegar poured over his ration at each feeding. The object of the apple cider vinegar, with its potassium and associated mineral content, was to create within the animal bodies the will for orderly growth and production of offspring.

The vinegar ration was started on November 1. By the last week in the following February each of the 23 cows had started a new pregnancy and in due time gave birth to a strong, vigorous calf which was on its feet within five minutes of birth and within a half-hour was nursing at the udder. Each calf had a heavy coat of hair and strong, rugged legs. Best of all, the calves were intelligent, bringing know-how across the bridge of life from their parents. It was not necessary to teach them to drink from a pail. They did so without teaching.

An equally interesting experience involved a kennel of boxer dogs. A dentist friend, raising the breed as a hobby and having a long waiting list of people who wanted to buy pups, told me that he had a serious problem in the fact that, though he had five bitches in the kennels, only one litter had been born in the last year.

On the folk medicine principle that this was due to a deficiency of potassium and other minerals, I suggested that once a day the ration of each dog be reinforced by one tablespoonful of apple cider vinegar.

At the end of one winter month he reported evidence that the apple cider vinegar had produced a chemical change in the dogs' bodies; their urine no longer stained snow yellow but left it white. During the following year all five bitches produced litters. The puppies were born strong and vigorous. It was affirmative normal completion of a pregnancy.

Earlier I made the point that laws which work with the animals will work just as well with humans. A medical-doctor friend lamented to me that no child had been born to him and his wife though they had been married seven years. They both desired a child very much but were beginning to resign themselves to a family life without children of their own. As they were both healthy individuals he was at a loss to account for this lack of children.

I suggested that he and his wife exchange wheat foods and wheat cereals for corn or oat cereals and corn or rye bread.

Instead of white sugar they used honey for sweetening food. They used such cold-climate fruits as apples, grapes and cranberries, all of which grow wild in Vermont, in place of citrus fruits such as oranges and grapefruit. At each meal he and his wife added two teaspoonfuls of honey and two teaspoonfuls of apple cider vinegar to a glass of water, sipping it during the meal as one would coffee or tea. As a result of this daily increase of potassium intake a pregnancy was started and in due time a strong, healthy child was born to the couple.

CHAPTER V

Your Racial Pattern and Vermont Folk Medicine

INTEREST IN DIFFERENT racial characteristics in humans is a natural part of Vermont folk medicine. It carries over from interest in the care and feeding of different breeds of cattle. Here in Vermont there are three head of cattle for every one person. A herd may be Holstein, Jersey, Guernsey, or some other breed. The farmer knows Guernseys and Holsteins cannot be identically fed, or Jerseys fed like some other breed. Of necessity he must learn the characteristics of the breed making up his dairy herd, in order to make his herd pay, for each cattle herd on a Vermont farm must show a profit.

As the farmer adapts the daily food intake to a specific breed of cattle, so Vermont folk medicine includes the theory that the individual should follow the food habits of his particular division of the race. By doing this a long step will be taken in prevention of sickness because the cells of the body will receive the kind of food they can use best.

We learn from plants that racial strain shows itself in physical characteristics. Take the cactus for example. We recognize cactus by certain features developed through countless generations. It has a natural immunity to heat, retains moisture, and thrives under environmental conditions its ancestors learned to combat and to use. For, say, a tomato plant or water cress, these conditions would not do at all.

In Europe the three white racial strains are Nordic, Alpine, and Mediterranean. The word Nordic means *northern.* The Nordics occupy the most northerly part, living in the north European coastal regions, which for several months of the year support no vegetation. Therefore Nordics are largely fish eaters, eating about ten times as much fish as meat. For vegetation, commonly land-grown elsewhere, they depend to a great extent on seaweed washed up on shore, and moss harvested from seacoast rocks.

The most striking physical characteristic of Nordics is blondness, a degree of blondness found in no other race. Nordics are generally tall, with blue, gray or green eyes, blond or light brown hair, narrow noses, very white skin, and long heads, by which is meant that the head measures more from front to back then from side to side.

The person living in a Nordic "human house" who is willing and able to follow the diet of his racial strain should find a newness of health, greater freedom from sickness, less dental decay, renewed energy. Wheat bread and wheat cereals will not be for you; your bread is rye bread. White sugar is not for you. Your proper sweetening agent is honey. Muscle meats are not for you. Instead of eating beef, lamb and pork, you should live out of the ocean, eating fish and other seafood. As for obtaining the values of Nordic vegetation, it is possible to buy seaweed tablets at health food, and drug, stores. They are generally called *kelp tablets.* The one I prescribe for patients is called Parkelp and is prepared by the Parkelp Company in San Pedro, California. The tablets include all of the forty-five different minerals which constitute kelp. One kelp tablet a day will provide the composite of minerals which the Nordic body has been conditioned through the centuries to receive.

You live in an Alpine "human house" if you have brown

or hazel eyes, chestnut brown or black hair, and a round head that has a tendency to breadth from ear to ear. Land-grown foods, such as cereals, and meat from game, flocks, and herds are for you.

If you have dark eyes, dark skin, black hair, and a long head, your "human house" is Mediterranean. You can eat all classes of food, such as seafood, dairy products, cereals, and fruit. Your system will especially favor corn cereals, grapes, and the juice of grapes.

All animals, including man, have the power to adapt themselves to surrounding conditions, but the adaptation is not accomplished in one or two generations, or even several. It must be recognized that in recent times a great change has taken place in the dietary habits of nearly all peoples. Development of machinery and transportation has made possible a tremendous increase of land under cultivation, hence in available food supply. This, in turn, has allowed a greatly expanded population, which grew the more rapidly because of advances made in control of epidemic disease. It has also changed the character of food from seafood to land-grown food. The change is especially drastic for those of Nordic descent.

The United States is a great proving ground of differences in the amount of essentials needed by different peoples. Here we have peoples of all racial strains living much the same as their neighbors within one or two generations. They buy their foods at the same stores and soon adopt the American way, losing the eating ways of their ancestors. After two or three generations the effects of a practically universal diet show differently in different peoples.

The difference in constituent requirements of kinds of crops is analogous to the different requirements of different people. Certain crops can be raised to advantage when the soil is new which cannot be raised later, when the soil has lost some of its constituents. Some farmers then turn to other crops whose mineral demands are of a different order. Eventually if the soil is mined instead of worked in this way, and lost minerals are not replaced, the soil will grow no crops profitably and one more is added to the thousands of deserted farms over the country.

The quantitative analyses of foods differ most in the mineral constituents. The difference lies mostly between land-grown and sea-grown foods. Through the leeching action of rainfall, much of the mineral matter of the land is washed into the sea. This applies especially to the more soluble minerals and their salts. The difference would be even greater, were it not for the fact that new soils are constantly being made by the disintegration of rock. Depletion is speeded up if crops are raised year after year without the replacement of minerals in the form of fertilizers.

Subdivisions of racial pattern are the anatomical pattern, the nervous, family (minus and plus), and the chemical patterns. Vermont folk medicine takes them all into account as helpful in understanding of the human machine.

By *anatomical pattern* I mean whether an individual is slender in build, of intermediate build, or stocky and broad in build.

In the slender type the whole bony framework of the body is light in form. As a whole the individual is either small and delicate, or tall and slender. As a rule the arms and legs are long, the face narrow. There is little excess fat. The skin is commonly soft and thin. There is an abundant growth of hair on the head; it is not easily lost, and often remains during the whole lifetime.

The intermediate type is often referred to as the *normal* type. The body figure is between the slender and heavy types.

The heavy type of body shows a build upon much sturdier lines. The bony framework is larger and heavier in structure. The muscles are large. The skin is thicker, as a rule, with less abundant growth of hair on the head. This hair is often lost early in life. Often too there is an excess of fat throughout the body. The neck is short and thick in proportion to the trunk, the shoulders are broad and square. As a whole the body is broad and relatively short. The chest is barrel-shaped, the arms and legs short. The face is broad and round.

Vermont folk medicine has gathered some interesting observations on the slender and heavy types of individual. Try to keep these in mind:

As a rule, if the slender type of individual becomes sick, it is in the spring of the year. Therefore that is the time when he should pay especially careful attention to his daily food intake. He should make sure to get sufficient sleep at night, and try to limit his daily activities. If he is in the habit of having a yearly medical checkup, he should have it in the spring.

On the other hand, if the heavy, broad, stocky type gets sick it is usually in the fall. He should observe the same precautions.

The heavy, broad type of individual shows greater wear during the later years of life than the slender type. In his younger days his human machine is very efficient and at its best. After the age of fifty it begins to show effects of wearing out.

On the other hand, the slender type may be a slow starter in life but he is an excellent finisher. Often he enjoys his best health after the age of fifty, and is pleasantly surprised at his endurance and sustained good health.

Blood pressure in the heavy type is generally higher than in the slender. Here in Vermont the blood pressure is generally higher during the cold months, when the body is trying to insulate itself against the cold by shifting the greater part of the blood from the skin to the interior of the body.

After looking at the body as a whole, it is helpful to study the size of the ear. Generally the individual with a large ear likes vegetables and bulky foods. The individual with a small ear prefers meat and more concentrated foods. Of course this is not invariably true, but it is true often enough to serve as a guide when advising a patient about his daily food intake in relation to returning him to his racial diet.

People living where they can observe domestic and wild animals learn in time that the nervous pattern in both animals and humans may be set by the parents. The establishment of this pattern lies in the daily food intake of both parents, especially the mother. One type of food intake will give a race-horse type of individual, while another type of food will produce a farm-horse type. Depending on the food intake, the new-born may be undersize or oversize. An otherwise excellent inheritance may be interrupted by wrong food selection, creating nutritional disaster.

The two divisions of the nervous system, designated as the *sympathetic* and the *parasympathetic,* may be likened to two gears with which one controls the power of a motor. By means of nutrition the parents have the determination whether the infant comes into the world with a dominant sympathetic division, which sets the human motor in high gear, or with a dominant parasympathetic division, which sets the human motor in low gear.

At a time of emergency, an assortment of changes go directly into service to make the body more effective. A violent display of energy is needed to meet the alarm; the human motor must shift into high gear. Among the changes are cessation of processes in the digestive tract; shifting of blood from the abdominal organs to the organs immediately essential to muscular exertion; increased vigor of contraction of the heart; discharge of extra blood corpuscles from the spleen; deeper breathing; dilation of the breathing tubes leading to the lungs; quick abolition of muscular fatigue; and mobilization of sugar in the circulation.

Lesser demands made on the nervous, endocrined, and chemical mechanisms in the body, which organize it for varying degrees of great effort, are made by fear, anxiety, unproductive worry, an unhappy environment, grief, a drop in outdoor temperature, and by certain foods. When day-by-day continuation of these factors maintain the body on one or another level of emergency organization, the body cells are denied the proper quantity of food they need to build up body reserves.

If you are one born into this world with your human motor set in high gear, Vermont folk medicine offers you help so that you may live your life with profit and pleasure to yourself. We in Vermont learn ways of shifting the human motor back to low gear or we would never be able, among other necessities, to withstand the characteristic and taxing weather changes of our environment.

The first of these helps has to do with your daily food intake. You should remove from it foods that produce an alkaline urine reaction. Such a reaction is produced when your human motor is set in high gear. You should bypass wheat foods and wheat cereals, instead using corn bread, corn muffins, pop corn, and canned corn. It is good practice to stay as close to corn as possible. You should use honey in place of white sugar. And, because here in Vermont oranges and grapefruit or their juices produce the unwanted alkaline urine reaction, you should instead use the juice or fruit of grapes, apples, and cranberries. Teach yourself to eat less meat and more fish and other seafood. Ocean-grown food acts as a sedative to your body. Notice how well you sleep at night after one or two lobsters were eaten at the evening meal.

You must provide for a daily intake of an organic acid, in order to combat the increased alkaline reaction of your blood brought about by the working of your human motor in high gear. On rising in the morning take two teaspoonfuls of apple cider vinegar in a glass of water, drinking it while dressing for breakfast.

Stay away from cold drinks, taking warm drinks instead. Try to remember that heat is a sedative to the body. There are a number of ways to get the heat your body needs—first, the sun bath if possible; or exposing the body to a lamp which gives out heat. A second way is to take a footbath, with enough hot water to cover feet and ankles. Allow the feet to remain in the hot water for 20 minutes. Do this at bedtime. The sedative effect will be shown in sound sleep. A third way is to place an electric pad between your back and the back of a chair, or across the abdomen until it has warmed the body. The last way is an electric blanket for sleeping.

Experimenting with methods used by Vermont folk medicine to shift the gears of your human motor, you will in time learn those which work best for you.

Two terms are used in relation to the family pattern.

The term *minus family pattern* is applied to an individual the majority of whose clinical data is below what is considered to be normal. The data are the pulse rate per minute, breathing rate per minute, temperature taken by mouth when free from disease, and blood pressure.

The term *plus family pattern* applies when all the clinical data taken by the doctor are normal.

No individual will represent either the minus or the plus family pattern 100 per cent. Usually the percentage will be about 75 per cent. If the findings fit the individual 60 to 80 per cent, it is considered satisfactory.

The minus pattern is traced as follows: In the earlier part of your life, up to twenty-five years, you were very energetic. You could start the day's work in early morning and continue till late at night without developing fatigue. If you attended a late party or dance you would not feel tired the following day. Your night's rest would bring you to the start of your new day feeling refreshed, ready and willing to do the day's work again. Others trying to work with and follow you would wonder whether you ever tired.

As the years passed, and you failed to follow your racial diet, a time came when you found yourself tired at the end of the day's work. The night's rest removed the sense of fatigue, enabling you to start fresh, but again you would be tired at the end of the day. Later still, a night's rest did not remove the sense of fatigue, and you found you started the next day a bit tired. As time went on, you found you were more or less tired all the time. The day's work ceased to give you pleasure. You lost your drive and initiative somewhat, and began to feel that a fairly long vacation of some kind was necessary in order for you to feel right again.

Now, though you tire physically, you never seem to tire mentally. If you sit down or lie down to rest, you grab a newspaper, magazine, or book to keep mentally employed. As a rule there is no lost mental time during the day. You are inclined to organize your life on a mental rather than a physical basis. Exercise outside of the physical activity required in your daily work is disappointing because it is apt to leave you tired instead of refreshed in body and mind. The day following physical exercise you are apt to find that you are dulled mentally.

For your minus family pattern the ideal exercise, if you feel the need, is gardening. The garden is never finished; hence it will hold your mental interest and satisfy your physical needs. What members of your family pattern need most is a mental house-cleaning, and it is best secured by one or more hobbies which do not require much physical activity. Music, stamp collecting, playing phonograph records or the radio, cards, books, auto trips, painting, drawing, crocheting, knitting, embroidery, or some one of the home crafts in wood or metal will bring an inner satisfaction that will return you to your day's work refreshed in mind and body. Members of this minus family pattern are very susceptible to a mental change. They often discover as the years pass that if they are feeling tired and mentally depressed an evening at the movie theater, reading an interesting book, watching television, a short auto ride, or time spent with an interesting hobby will produce as much refreshment as physical exercise produces for people of the opposite family pattern.

When you feel right you sleep soundly. Noises in the house, thunder in the heavens, cars passing in the street will not wake you. When you do not feel right, you sleep lightly. It is easy for you to wake up between midnight and 3:00 A.M. and not easy to fall asleep again.

From six to ten o'clock in the morning is a more difficult time for you than from six to ten in the evening. When bedtime comes you are often wide awake, feel at your best, and want to sit up rather than go to bed. You are apt to wake up in the morning with a mean-feeling head but the feeling will generally wear off by mid-morning. If it does not, but becomes a real headache, that day is spoiled for you and you try to sidestep as much of the day's work as possible. You may find you are troubled at times by a headache in the back part of your head and a feeling of tightness in the back of your neck. At times you are bothered by an itching head, which may be relieved by a shampoo. You are apt to be annoyed by an itching of the nose, causing you to rub it continually to stop the itching. Your skin will itch and may range all the way from requiring an occasional scratching to obliging you to leave the room so that you can give your body a good scratching in private.

You are troubled by cold hands and feet. It is easy for your feet and hands to go to sleep. If you cross your knees it is very easy for a foot to go to sleep. It is not uncommon for the type you represent to wake up during the night with numb hands if you sleep with your arms crossed, making it necessary to chafe the hands in order to restore feeling in them. At times you may be annoyed by aching arms and legs.

You do not enjoy extremes of temperature. In cold weather you do not care to go outdoors any more than is absolutely necessary, for it is difficult for your body to adapt to low temperature. If you do go out you take great care to have your feet and hands covered warmly in order not to feel miserable, as you do if your hands or feet become cold. On the other hand, when the thermometer soars during the summer months, reaching a reading of ninety degrees or more, you "flat-tire" and have no ambition to work. You feel best when the temperature is either moderately warm or moderately cold. If you were obliged to choose between very hot and very cold weather, I should expect you to choose cold, because of the two you feel better in cold than in hot weather.

You do not enjoy extremes of temperature in your food either. While some members of your family pattern do enjoy hot foods, generally the majority like their food warm. It is not satisfying when cold. In a restaurant, if a plate of hot soup is placed before you, you are apt to wait for it to cool a bit.

While you can eat foods direct from the refrigerator, as a rule you don't care to. You eat ice cream slowly, taking longer than others to eat the same amount; you like to warm it up in your mouth before swallowing it. While you can drink ice water you prefer drinking water only as cold as it will come from the tap.

While you do not have many colds, any that you do have are apt to go down into your chest and last a long time. When you are tired the resonance goes out of your voice. You discover you are obliged to put more effort into talking, in order for your voice to sound to you as it usually does. Those who know you well can tell when you are tired, for your voice sounds dull to them.

Members of your family pattern often believe that they are inclined to be bilious because they have dizzy spells at times, and there is often an uncomfortable sensation on the right side just above the waist line. For no apparent reason you are apt to belch gas after eating. At other times there is a burning sensation in the stomach about an hour after eating. Occasionally you have a feeling of abdominal distention, finding it necessary to loosen the clothing around your waist line. Unless you have disciplined yourself to a specific time for the daily bowel movement, you are probably troubled with constipation.

If the medical men you have consulted from time to time have been interested in operating, you probably had one or more of four operations done: on your nose, removal of your tonsils, removal of your appendix, and an operation on your gall bladder.

As a rule, members of your family pattern live a long time, generally beyond eighty years of age. Probably in your family tree one or more individuals lived to be ninety years or over.

All in all, you have good days and poor days, with a larger number of poor days. When you have a good day you feel wonderful, and you ponder what needs to be done in order to feel right all the time.

If you are a minus family pattern individual, a number of observations relating to your food should interest you.

White sugar does not give you the energy you so much need to do the day's work. If you will change to honey, you will find that it gives you that needed energy. Apparently you are able to handle a balanced sugar as represented by honey, but not the sugar from which the values have been removed in refining. Too, honey does not have to be digested in the human body; this has already been done in the stomach of the honey bee. Four to six teaspoonfuls of honey a day, divided among the different meals, should be enough. You will notice that you are less nervous and that you sleep better at night. Honey is a mild laxative, and if you should be taking too much because you like it you will note its laxative action on your bowels. Regulate the amount you take.

You just don't handle white flour well, so it is not for you. It generally makes you stomach-conscious, being very apt to produce gas in your stomach, often heartburn after eating, and constipation. The effect on you will be to upset the timetable of your digestive tract. Generally you handle corn and rye foods well, so your breads should be corn or rye. On the whole, as you study yourself, you will note that you do not digest cereals any too well.

You need to study your protein intake, represented by the muscle meats, milk, eggs, nuts, legumes, fowl, fish, and seafood. Protein food is designed by Nature to repair the wear and tear on body tissue brought about by a day's work. There is no provision for storing protein in the human body as there is for storing fat and sugar. Because of this lack of storage facilities, the excess of protein not needed for the repair of body tissues must be eliminated from the body.

If a catarrhal discharge is present in your breathing tract; if you are subject to frequent head colds, occasional bronchitis attacks, or influenza; or if you have sinus trouble or sometimes pneumonia, then you should reappraise your daily intake of protein food. You can render your body susceptible to these various sicknesses any time you eat from day to day a high protein-low vegetable and fruit diet. Take an illustration from the garden. In growing plants, one has to avoid the addition of too much nitrogen to the soil; too much nitrogen increases the amount of plant disease in the garden. In the human body protein food is the source of nitrogen. Too much protein food leads to human sickness as well as to plant and animal sickness.

Vegetables and fruit, nuts and legumes are for the minus family pattern individual. In addition to those, he gets along very well with fish and other seafood.

As far as the biochemical make-up of the minus family pattern individual is concerned, his greatest problem is calcium metabolism. If this is lower than it should be, he observes that, as a child, he does not grow as well as he should. Decay of the teeth is apt to be present; the hair combs out more than it should, the fingernails break or tear easily.

The compound in the body which forms bones, teeth, hair, and fingernails consists of ten parts calcium and four parts phosphorus. Generally the needed phosphorus is present. It is the ten parts calcium that are less than should be.

Raise the blood calcium by taking honey. Blood studies show that the blood calcium will rise two and one-half hours after honey is taken, and will stay up for twenty-four hours. Honey taken each day will maintain the ten parts of calcium needed to unite with the four parts of phosphorus.

If you are of the plus family pattern, generally you are physically strong.

In youth this type of individual is very active physically, engaging in athletic games, contests, and all outdoor and indoor sports. He is fond of hiking, fishing, hunting, golf, tennis. For him life's best expression is physical rather than mental.

As he grows up he is seldom sick if he is able to exercise and avoid too much indoor life. The appetite generally is good, with a fondness for meat, pastry, and sweets. Banquets, annual feasts such as Thanksgiving and Christmas, class dinners, and the like are greatly enjoyed. As a rule, this person does not care for vegetables and salads.

If by circumstance a member of this plus family pattern is compelled to spend most of the time indoors, because his life is organized on a mental basis, then sooner or later he is apt to find that he is tired all the time. Instead of being a joy, the day's work represents a dull round of daily duties to be got through somehow. He is irritable when he does not wish to be. He is a bit hard to live with when that is the last thing he wishes to be. He goes about with a hair-trigger type of disposition and is easily offended by others. He blows up frequently and is prone to bawl out people. During the middle of the day, when he should be most awake, he is drowsy. When bedtime comes he often finds it difficult to fall asleep. His night's rest brings him only moderate refreshment, and he comes to the beginning of a new day a bit tired. From six to ten o'clock in the morning is easier for him to get through than from six to ten in the evening. He has vague symptoms of short duration in various parts of the body. He is subject to constipation. His skin inclines to dryness. His hair comes out a bit more than he would wish. All in all a long vacation of some sort seems to him his only chance to feel right again.

As with individuals of the minus family pattern, there are findings relative to food which should interest the person belonging to the plus family pattern.

Honey should be used because the nervous system of this type is very apt to become overactive. Honey, being sedative to the body, will calm it down. Each day six teaspoonfuls of strained honey should be apportioned among the day's meals.

In your most physically active years your system can better handle the protein foods—muscle meats, milk, eggs, nuts, legumes such as peas and beans, fowl, fish, and seafood. As you reach the age of forty you will need to review your daily food intake. In order to prevent undesirable effects on the body as you become physically less active, the protein intake should be lessened.

You should also understand your chemical pattern.

It is possible to influence the chemical pattern of an animal or human being in much the same manner as we may influence the nervous pattern. If you follow radio and television you constantly hear the terms *acid* and *alkaline.*

Sodium in the blood enables it to maintain a normal, weakly alkaline reaction by neutralizing an excess of acid coming to it from the activity of the body cells as they burn food intake and from the use of the body muscles in work or play. In their vital activity, body cells manufacture lactic acid, carbonic acid, phosphoric acid, and sulfuric acid.

The mechanism which regulates the body's chemical balance between acid and alkaline consists mainly of the blood, lungs, and kidneys. When the secretion of acid in the stomach is at its height, directly after a meal, the blood is more alkaline. The kidneys, being spill-over organs used by the blood to rid itself of material it does not wish to keep, allow the sodium to pass through them, with the result that the urine changes from its normal acid reaction to an alkaline reaction. Later, when food leaves the stomach and enters the bowels, it is absorbed into the blood stream, and as the acid reaches the blood the sodium content of the blood is lowered. Now the blood wishes to get rid of the acid. As the acid passes through the kidneys it returns the urine to its normal acid reaction.

The lungs represent another means by which the blood may get rid of acid. Blood, when flowing through the lungs, gives off carbonic acid, which helps the blood to maintain its normal weakly alkaline reaction.

We speak of the body "organizing for fight or flight," meaning the diverse effects of emotion. With reference to this, let us consider the relation of the emotion of fear to the urine reaction, as observed when taken with Squibb's Nitrazine Paper, on rising in the morning, and before the evening meal. Squibb's Nitrazine Paper is a specially prepared paper which turns yellow if the urine reaction is acid, and blue if it is alkaline. You can purchase this paper by the bottle of 100 strips at any drugstore.

I use as an example three "human guinea pigs" who had consistently been showing an acid urine reaction, when specimens were taken on rising and before the evening meal, which suddenly shifted to an alkaline urine reaction. They were members of one family: father, mother, and a married son living nearby.

Efforts to trace down the cause of this shift brought to light the information that a second son would go on occasional drinking parties, usually ending up by his being brought home intoxicated. The family was socially prominent, and these incidents were completely upsetting. While one brother was out looking for the troublesome member of the family, father and mother waited at home in fear and anxiety. It was the fear and anxiety which brought the shift over to the alkaline urine reaction.

This relation of fear to an alkaline urine reaction has been observed in many other individuals. For example, a farm woman, sixty-two years of age, consistently showed an acid urine reaction. Suddenly a urine reaction form brought to the office during the month of February showed an alkaline urine for a period of two weeks. We sought the explanation.

It seems that, owing to unusually cold weather, the farm water-supply system, which connected with a spring, began showing signs of freezing, with the prospect of a stoppage in the flow of water. If this happened it meant that water for the house and the farm animals had to be fetched from a brook two miles distant, a hard and time-consuming job in below-zero weather. This had already happened once a number of years earlier. If the complication of a severe snow-storm should be added, it would be extremely difficult to supply the dairy herd with needed water.

Fear over the farm water supply had caused a shift of the urine reaction from acid to alkaline. As soon as the weather modified and the danger of the water supply freezing had passed, the urine reaction returned to acid.

A patient in her early sixties was known throughout Vermont as a singer of Vermont folk songs, learned in childhood days and now sung from time to time in public. Each August there was a state convention for the preservation of old-time music and dancing, and the patient, who had been running a steadily acid urine reaction, suddenly ran an alkaline reaction for three days. She was questioned as to her specific activities during those three days and it turned out that she had been scared that she would forget the words of her songs. As soon as the folk festival was behind her, the urine reaction returned to normal.

Food will have a pronounced effect in determining acidity or alkalinity of urine reaction. The low-protein high-carbohydrate daily food intake recommended by Nature organizes the body for peace and quiet, enabling the body to build up and store body reserves against time of need. But when man rearranges Nature's plans to suit his own desires, placing food emphasis on protein instead of carbohydrates, he is organizing his body for fight and flight.

These are no sometime-rules. If human or animal parents live under conditions which arouse the emotions, and eat a high protein-low carbohydrate diet, the baby will be born into this world exhausted from combating an existence of fight and flight while it is within the mother's body, trying to build a body. In other words, an otherwise excellent inheritance is spoiled by the parents' trying to rearrange Nature's plan. This interrupted inheritance may, and certainly will, affect the brain, muscle system, digestive tract, nervous system, and the size of the newborn. It will be undersized and underweight. It may have unexpected markings. It will not be as mentally alert as it should be. Coordination between brain and muscle will be below normal. Coming into the world with a body organized for fight and flight instead of for peace and quiet, it will start off with less chance of building up needed body reserves. The sodium content of its blood is too high, the urine reaction most often alkaline, not normally acid. If protected and encouraged it may manage to make its way in life, but generally it lacks the endurance needed for success. Sickness comes often to such a body. All in all it experiences difficulty in adjusting itself to its environment.

Take an example from the animal world. When Nature's plan of excellent inheritance is interrupted in hunting dogs, the young dogs are timid. When training them to hunt birds it is necessary to cajole and encourage them. Young dogs whose excellent inheritance is upheld by right diet before and after birth are, on the contrary, bold. It will often be necessary to call them during training, for they will be too eager.

In cattle, even after superior breeding, when an excellent

inheritance is marred by wrong diet, a calf will be weak and fussy. It will not get up quickly after being born, as it should. It will be lacking in intelligence and alertness. It will have to be taught to drink out of a pail. When it takes its place in the herd it cannot be worked hard and is one of the first to become sick. Its milk production will be poor in the light of expectations from the superior breeding of its parents.

Conversely, if diet preparation has been what it should be the calf will come into the world at its proper size. It will have a heavy coat of hair and strong rugged legs. Five minutes after it is born it will be on its feet, and in a half hour nursing at the udder. It will not regard a pail as a mystery but will drink out of it at once. Joining the herd it will, as the saying goes, "be a credit to its folks."

The explanation, whether in animals or humans, is that interrupted inheritance produces a change of chemical pattern which, in turn, makes adjustment as an individual to its environment difficult—perhaps, for all practical purposes, impossible.

What can we do to provide against this?

Let us take hunting dogs as an example. We want no abortion. We want a normal number of pups in a litter. We want pups strong at birth, with a supply of body reserves enabling them to develop well.

We ensure this by adding to the mother's one ration per day one tablespoonful of apple cider vinegar. This brings over everything that was in the apple originally except the change that takes place in the sugar content of the apple juice. What we are after in the apple is the potassium, which organizes the body for peace and quiet and the building and storing of body reserves. Thus are we able to help the mother build a pup-body incorporating the right chemical, nervous, and anatomical patterns.

Throughout the pregnancy of a cow two ounces of apple cider vinegar are poured over the twice-daily feeding ration when it is placed in the feed trough. This is continued each

day until the calf is born. During the last three months of
her pregnancy, on Monday, Wednesday and Friday of each
week, three drops of Lugol's solution of iodine—5 per cent
elemental iodine in 10 per cent solution of potassium
iodide—are added to the apple cider vinegar.

The human expectant mother should take the following
throughout pregnancy: on rising in the morning, one teaspoonful of apple cider vinegar in a glass of water, taken
while dressing. At one meal during the day, two teaspoonfuls
of apple cider vinegar and two teaspoonfuls of honey in a
glass of water, taken during the meal as one would take a
cup of coffee or tea.

During the last three months of pregnancy, on Tuesday
and Friday of each week, to this is added one drop of Lugol's
solution of iodine.

This program, combined with the previously noted ex-
changing of wheat foods and cereals for rye and corn foods,
honey in place of white sugar, and so forth, should establish
for the infant an excellent chemical pattern with which to
meet its new environment. As it grows toward adult life
beneficial results of the pattern will be seen in sustained
good health and easy adjustment to environmental changes.

CHAPTER VI

The First Yardstick of Your Health

THE FIRST YARDSTICK of your health is the urine. Vermont folk medicine believes that sickness appears on an alkaline-urine background.

To study whether sickness appears in human beings on an alkaline or acid urine background, I set up tests with the cooperation of twelve children five years or under in age, and twelve adults. For two years these twenty-four human guinea pigs kept a daily urine-reaction record and a daily record of food taken at each day's three meals. They came to my office every two weeks for a check-up and to report their records. Each time temperature, pulse, breathing rate, and blood pressure were taken. The color of the nasal mucous membrane was observed, the throat studied, and the presence and appearance of lymphoid tissue in the throat noted. In addition to the urine-reaction records and food diary, continuing study was made of the number of daily bowel movements, the number of times urine was passed in each twenty-four-hour period, the number of hours of sleep at night, and whether sleep was sound, fairly sound, or restless.

It soon appeared that fluctuations in urine reaction took place in relation to meals. In their book *Acidosis and Alkalosis,* Graham and Morris describe this as follows:

42

About one hour before breakfast there is a rise in the bicarbonate of the blood, which is the result of the loss of chlorine secreted in the gastric juice. Simultaneously the urine becomes more alkaline. This phenomenon is known as the "alkaline tide" and is most marked in patients with hyperchlorhydria, and absent in those with achlorhydria. When the food has passed into the intestine and reabsorption of the chlorine of the gastric juice is taking place, the bicarbonate and chlorine of the blood regain their normal levels, and the urinary reaction returns to its usual acidity.*

In time it became clear that the reaction of the urine passed on rising in the morning gives the greatest amount of information, because of the length of time represented by the night's sleep. The next best time to take the urine reaction is just before the evening meal. The reaction of the morning urine shows whether the night's sleep was sufficient to establish the normal acid reaction. The reaction taken before the evening meal shows to what degree the day's activities have influenced it. If it still remains acid, then all is well; but if it has shifted to alkaline, then the reason must be sought.

The first observation made of these subjects related to the common cold. It appeared that when a common cold was on the way the urine reaction shifted to alkaline, continuing alkaline for several days in advance of the appearance of the cold. During recovery from the cold the urine reaction shifted back to acid and continued so. It was possible to induce recovery from the common cold by shifting the urine reaction to the acid side.

It was observed that the urine reaction shifted from acid to alkaline before the onset of one of the childhood diseases such as chicken pox or measles. When therapeutic measures capable of shifting the urine back to the acid side were used, the childhood disease either did not appear at all or it appeared in only mild form, with rapid recovery.

* Stanley Graham, M.D., and Noah Morris, M.D., *Acidosis and Alkalosis* (Edinburgh, E. & S. Livingstone, 1933), p. 48.

Patients were studied from the viewpoint of the relation of their clinical condition to their urine reaction. It was learned in time that paranasal sinusitis was associated with the alkaline urine reaction. In one subject to attacks of paranasal sinusitis the alkaline reaction could be observed for from one to two weeks before the actual attack appeared. As with the childhood diseases, if measures were taken to shift the urine reaction to the acid side the attacks either did not come on at all or were mild, and recovery rapid.

A connection was observed between symptoms of asthma and the alkaline urine reaction. Hay fever and many other clinical conditions showed the same connection, the same characteristic improvement with shifting of the reaction to the acid side.

By the end of the two years it was possible to answer the original question: "Does sickness come when the urine reaction is alkaline or when it is acid?" The answer is that sickness comes when the reaction, taken at the two best daily junctures with Squibb's Nitrazine Paper, is alkaline, the paper turning blue.

The relation of clinical conditions to an alkaline urine reaction leads one to suspect that in different individuals there exist different biochemical targets in different parts of the body. When one of these targets is hit, an alarm reaction appears in the form of symptoms. Since the underlying cause is the same, regardless of which target is hit, treatment is similar. The importance of making a diagnosis is thus lessened, for the indication is to restore to normal the chemistry and physiology of the body.

The second urine observation relates to the weather. It was noted that two days before a drop in weather temperature the urine reaction shifted to the alkaline side, requiring one to two days to adjust to the normal acid reaction after the weather change actually appeared. In winter, when mothers of the children being studied noticed the connection between the drop in weather temperature and a shift in the children's urine to the alkaline side, they began keeping the windows closed in the children's sleeping rooms. Inviting an alkaline urine by keeping the window open in cold weather was to invite an onset of sickness. Keeping the window closed helped materially in maintaining an acid urine, thus avoiding sicknesses heralded by the alkaline evidence.

The question naturally arose, If cold shifts the urine reaction to alkaline, will heat shift the urine reaction back to acid? Our study subjects were asked to work out the answer.

It was found that a hot bath would shift urine, become alkaline, back to acid. With this evidence at hand, the bowl of hot lemonade sipped slowly and the hot foot bath, which mothers have learned from Vermont folk medicine to depend on when a child appears to be coming down with some sickness, began to make medical sense.

I found substantiation of this evidence in the course of visiting a medical friend in the Middle West. This friend mentioned that he was in the habit of taking a Turkish bath when he felt physically fatigued, and found that it had a relieving effect. I asked if he would be willing to test his urine with Squibb's Nitrazine Paper before and after the Turkish bath, and he agreed immediately. Later he reported to me that just before the bath was taken the urine showed evidence of the fatigue by its alkalinity, whereas after the bath the shift to acid appeared. Clearly, the heat of the bath had brought about the chemical change in the body.

This gave me the idea of asking my twenty-four human guinea pigs to test effects of physical fatigue on the urine reaction. From the reports it was evident that the circumstances under which the fatigue developed made a difference in the urine reaction. One adult showed by his daily urine reactions that, any time he ran an alkaline urine reaction, a half day of hunting in the woods would shift him back to the acid side. If, on the other hand, he worked around home, the urine would still be alkaline in reaction. This was supported by the report of another adult who said that if he did such physical work as cleaning out the garage his urine reaction would shift to alkaline; but that if he spent Sunday afternoon skiing on the mountainside, his urine reaction would remain acid or, if it had been alkaline before skiing, would shift to acid.

If hard physical work unconnected with sport or recreation produced an alkaline urine reaction, the question arose as to what effect mental work had on the urine reaction. Included among my twelve adult subjects were five mental workers; with their cooperation it was possible to work out the observation that prolonged mental work produces an alkaline urine reaction.

If we lose our childhood instincts for selecting foods best suited to the needs of body chemistry and physiology at the moment, we deprive ourselves of a significant help in maintaining health. Let us consider, then, whether the urine reaction may serve as a substitute for our discarded instincts, helping us to select the right daily food intake. In due time, with the help of these human guinea pigs, a food list was worked out of items which, here in Vermont, produce the alkaline reaction. The first of these was wheat, in the form of bread, cake, crackers, cookies, doughnuts and wheat cereals if taken as daily food.

Another food observation was that whereas white, brown, and maple sugar and maple syrup produced an alkaline urine reaction, honey will not do so. A number of individuals living on farms having maple-sugar orchards were asked to study their urine reaction before, during, and after the maple-sugar season. This study showed that both maple sugar and maple syrup produced an alkaline urine reaction in individuals who, previous to taking them, had showed a daily acid urine reaction record. With the result of this observation at hand, I could understand why sour pickles, preserved in vinegar, always were served with maple-sugar-on-snow. Evidently it was part of Vermont folk medicine that the vinegar in the pickles, which produces an acid urine reaction, offset the ill effects of the maple sugar in producing an alkaline urine reaction.

It is manifestly not possible within the confines of this book to go into all the studies made in relation to urine reaction. But before going on, having observed its relation to development of sickness, the weather, food, and physical and mental fatigue, we ought to consider the urine reaction to pain.

The pain of paranasal sinusitis is associated with an alkaline urine reaction. As a rule one can shift the reaction to acid, relieving the pain, by taking one teaspoonful of apple cider vinegar in a glass of water each hour for seven doses.

The pain of facial neuralgia is also associated with an alkaline urine reaction. The same proportion of apple cider vinegar to water, taken every hour, will usually relieve this pain because the urine reaction will have been shifted to acid. Instead of drinking down the entire contents of the glass of acidified water at one time, it often works best to sip them.

All acids do not produce the same effect in the body. For example, dilute hydrochloric acid in five to ten drop doses in a glass of water four times a day for a period of two weeks will *increase* the pain of arthritis of the small joints of the hands and feet, whereas one teaspoonful of apple cider vinegar in a glass of water four times a day will result in marked relief of the pain in the same period of time.

As said at the beginning of this chapter, the urine reaction is the first yardstick of health. These studies therefore made an extremely enlightening basis for continuing studies in other directions.

CHAPTER **VII**

The Instincts of Childhood

THERE ARE SELF-PROTECTIVE instincts in young children which impel them to seek foods needed at the moment by their body cells.

I made a study of children under ten years of age who lived on Vermont farms, in order that I might learn the workings of these instincts. I discovered that these young farm children chewed cornstalks, ate raw potatoes, raw carrots, raw peas, raw string beans, raw rhubarb, berries, green apples, ripe apples, the grapes that grow wild throughout the state, sorrel, timothy grass heads, and the part of the timothy stem that grows underground. They ate salt from the cattle box, drank water from the cattle trough, chewed hay, ate calf food and, by the handful, a dairy-ration supplement containing seaweed; they even filled their pockets with this, to eat during school.

There was an opportunity also to study some children from a nearby village. For several years I studied a herd of 45 registered Jersey cows. The owner of the farm loved children, and the children came from the village to his farm to play in the hay, ride the farm horses when they were in the pasture, feed the hens, collect the eggs, and feed the calves.

A pail of apple cider vinegar went on the feed car, with a cup to measure out what was poured over the cows' ration.

When the children discovered the vinegar they would take a dip of it in the cup and drink it. They would also drink it from the pail in the barn, just as it came from the vinegar barrel. When I had watched them for a while, I estimated that during the day each child would consume from one to two ounces. I learned also that at meals, when apple cider vinegar was poured over sliced cucumbers, they would lick every last drop from the saucer.

It is not absolutely clear why young children like sour drinks, but they do. Their favorite, I have observed, is cranberry juice. It is not necessarily because its beautiful red color has a powerful eye appeal, for I have often seen them drink it from thick china cups, with little of the color showing. I have heard it suggested that children's favorite is cranberry juice because cranberries mean Christmas to them.

The only certain thing is that they like sour drinks. The cranberry juice, which contains four acids, they will drink so sour that an adult would not touch it. In my part of Vermont during the summer months they will go about looking for rhubarb stalks to break off and chew. They eat the acid leaves of sorrel, which is one of the sourest of the perennial herbs. Some deep instinct drives them to seek kinds of food needed for body building, namely a high-carbohydrate, low-protein food intake, which is acid in reaction before it enters the mouth. If we were wise enough to carry over into adult life the instincts of childhood, we would make a point of eating fruit, berries, edible leaves, and edible roots that would not be cooked.

Among Vermonters who live close to the soil, I have found many who do this. I learned that they eat the following:

Beechnut-tree leaves, which taste sour.
Maple-tree leaves, which at first taste sour but then change to a sweet taste.
Elm-tree leaves, which have a neutral taste but quickly relieve the sensation of hunger. In fact, of all tree leaves, they are the quickest and best in relieving hunger.

Willow-tree leaves, which taste sour.

Apple-tree leaves, which taste bitter.

Chokecherry-tree leaves, which taste a little sour, like a cherry drink at the drugstore.

Poplar-tree leaves, which taste bitter, but not as bitter as the leaves of the apple tree.

Birch-tree leaves.

The bush whose tender leaves Vermont farm people eat as a matter of course is the raspberry bush. The leaves are commonly eaten by both men and women.

Native Vermonters have been aware for generations of the value and flavor of the tender young leaves of plants that grow wild in abundance in the woods, and habitually gather and eat them. When cultivated greens are very scarce in the springtime, the first wild green leaves are eagerly sought, out of craving for the fresh green flavor and nutritive qualities lacking in the winter meals.

These wild leaves belong very definitely to the protective-foods group. Besides their food value, their appetizing flavor, color, and crispness make foods with which they are served more interesting. Most of the wild greens are at their best in spring and early summer, before cultivated varieties are ready for use. There are any number of plants native to Vermont that are to be found in many other sections, and that are not only appetizing, cooked or uncooked, in salads, but are extremely rich in the properties on which folk medicine is based. Some are only found growing wild while others are plants which may be found in gardens or other areas under cultivation. To identify some of them, their character and use:

Marsh marigold, or cowslip, grows, as the name indicates, in marshes, moist meadows, and swampy areas. The leaves are cooked.

Fern tops, when just out of the ground, and before they un-roll. These fiddle-tops, or fiddleheads as they are also sometimes called because of their resemblance to the neck of a violin, are the curled young fronds of the cinnamon fern. They grow in damp places, often along the roadside, and are picked when they are young and tender. They grow in clusters and have dark green, smooth, shiny stems, with a brown cap over the fuzzy fiddlehead. They may be cooked like any other green or used raw in a salad. They taste like asparagus and in Vermont are regarded as delicious.

Horseradish leaves are cooked for eating.

As elsewhere, dandelions are plentiful in Vermont. They are willing to grow almost anywhere, in fields, meadows, by the roadside, on lawns around the house. The best time to gather them for eating purposes is in the spring and early summer before they become tough and very bitter. They are cut below the ground so that a section of the root remains attached to the leaves. The young tender plants in the spring are best raw in salads. When they are a little older, they taste better cooked.

Dock is a leafy plant, to be used raw in salads, cooked as a green by itself, or in combination with other plants. It is common in both cultivated and waste land. Frequently it is found in hayfields after a new seeding.

The yellow rocket cress is a common weed found in both waste and cultivated land, in meadows, along streams and roadsides, and in fields. In the spring the crown of the rosette of leaves is used before the yellow flowers appear. This may be eaten either raw or cooked.

Water cress grows in Vermont along the margins of brooks. Its best seasons are spring and autumn. Because of its flavor the water cress gives zest to almost any salad or sandwich.

Many people do not know that the common milkweed is an edible plant. Milkweed plants are found in abundance along almost every country road, and also in open fields and the meadows. They should be used only when young, while stems are tender. The young leaves make a good cooked green, and the new young shoots are excellent when cooked like asparagus.

The tender top of the plant is eaten raw and tastes like green peas fresh out of the garden.

Pigweed is a common wasteland weed, often found also in cultivated fields and gardens. It grows to a height of about five feet. The stems and lower surfaces of the leaves are characterized by a mealy-white covering. The leaves are cooked like spinach.

The mustard plant is a weed which is very tasty, cooked separately or in combination with other greens. The tender young leaves add flavor to salads. It is recognized by its rough, hairy leaves.

Purslane is another abundant weed, found in both wasteland and cultivated areas. It thrives in hot weather and produces small yellow flowers. It is one of the most delicious of the wild greens, is very simple to gather and prepare, and may be eaten raw or cooked like spinach.

Children are not the only ones who favor sorrel. Garden sorrel, found in neglected fields and grasslands, and sometimes even in cultivated areas, is relished by adults, who like it either cooked or raw. It is often used in sandwiches, like water cress.

Checkerberry leaves are eaten raw.

A number of the green vegetables whose leaves are used as foods are found in Vermont gardens. These include not only greens for cooking but also the salad leaves, usually served uncooked in the salad bowl.

Lettuce heads the list of these green leaves.

Endive is next in importance. It comes in two types, broad-leaved and curly-leaved, and both have a flavor which is distinctive.

Corn-salad leaves have a fresh and spicy flavor which makes them a welcome ingredient for the salad bowl.

Curled garden cress thrives with ordinary garden culture, and contributes a pungent flavor to salads.

Chervil is an aromatic plant, somewhat resembling parsley but superior in flavor; it is used both in salad bowls and to garnish meats.

Chives are a most useful salad vegetable. They are a cousin of the onion, the leaves have a delicate oniony flavor, just enough to season a salad. They bear an attractive lavender flower and are often used as a border along the garden path.

Turnip top leaves are cooked for eating, spinach leaves used either cooked or raw, cabbage leaves also. Parsley is used as a food during the months when it is in the garden; in the fall, one or more parsley plants are transferred by Vermonters to a flower pot and grown indoors through the winter for food use.

A number of leaves used as food are classified by native Vermonters as herbs. Some grow wild in fields and woods; many may be grown in the garden. Herbs are at their best when fresh but are satisfactory also when dried. There are many ways to use herbs in cooking. Here in Vermont as elsewhere, certain herbs have come to be immediately associated with certain foods, such as mint with lamb, dill with pickles, caraway in cookies, basil with tomatoes, and savory with string beans. Several of the herbs are particularly good in salads.

Anise leaves are a hardy annual in Vermont. The leaves are lacy, and there are white flowers. Anise leaves are used in flavoring salads.

The common basil is a shrubbery plant about a foot in height. The leaves and flowers have a clovelike, spicy flavor and are prized for seasoning soups, meats, and salads and for flavoring tomato cookery. The harvesting time is when the plants are in bloom. The tender tips are cut with their foliage, tied in small bunches, and dried for winter use.

Borage leaves, a rough-stemmed, leafy annual in Vermont, are cooked and served like spinach. The plant bears flowers of a lovely blue.

Burnet leaves come from the garden burnet, a hardy perennial herb with mats of long compound leaves; the portion of the plant used is the young leaf which grows from the almost ever-green mats all winter; used in salad the leaves give a distinctive flavor resembling cucumbers.

Caraway leaves are used in salads, with the young shoots. The plant grows about two feet in height and often is found growing wild.

We are all familiar with using celery leaves for flavor in soups, stews and salads.

The leaves of the sweet cicely plant are fernlike and used in cooking.

Dill and fennel are good for seasoning.

Although the rose geranium is commonly regarded as a house plant for decoration, the leaves, used in cooking, impart a rose flavor. One of its commonest uses is the flavoring of apple jelly; the leaves are used also to flavor puddings and custards.

Horehound leaves are dried and used in Vermont to make a tea used in treating the common cold.

Peppermint grows in Vermont beside the brooks. The leaves are eaten commonly by native Vermonters and chopped pepper-mint leaves are found in small cans for a few pennies in Barre grocery stores.

The nasturtium is an annual, grown in the flower garden. The leaves have a peppery taste, and Vermonters use them in sand-wiches and salads.

Rosemary, sage, savory, spearmint, tarragon, burdock and wintergreen leaves are all in common use. Aside from their virtues in varying the flavors of foods, they are important for their mineral and other values.

Adding up all the various plant leaves and those growing on trees and bushes, we find we have 53 varieties of leaves that are regularly eaten by the native Vermonter living close to the soil.

A number of leaves which are alterative, antiseptic, and mildly diuretic are sold in drugstores for making herb teas. These leaves are prepared as an infusion by steeping one ounce to one pint of boiling water; cook and strain. The adult dose is a half-teacupful two or three times a day. A tea made from catnip leaves is often used. It is very acid in reaction. Mullein leaves, used for coughs, colds, diarrhea, and so on, are a demulcent, a diuretic, and an anodyne. Pennyroyal leaves furnish an aromatic stimulant which is useful in relieving colic; the dose, one wineglassful of infusion. Plantain leaves are also very good, medically speaking, as an infusion.

I discussed these different leaves with a medical friend who had been born in Vermont and raised on a farm. After reading over the list of leaves obtained from trees, bushes, and plants, he said that he had eaten practically all of them when he lived on the farm.

It is quite evident from a study of the edible leaves eaten by the native Vermonter who lives close to the soil that the leaves which play such an important part in the daily food intake are eaten from instinct. If you have carried over your childhood instincts into your adult life, you will be one of those people fond of leafy salads, and you will have demonstrated to yourself many times that they bear a definite relation to your continued well-being. Your body, designed for the living of primitive times, expects to receive a daily intake of leaves. In these more civilized times the body still needs these leaves as much as ever, in order to better stand the stress and strain of modern living. If you have not formed the habit, it is never too late to begin to add leafy salads to your daily food intake.

CHAPTER VIII

Potassium and Its Uses

THE MORE ONE OBSERVES that the principles and applications of Vermont folk medicine are interchangeable among all living things, the more one is impressed by the underlying importance of potassium as a common treatment agent. The different remedies prescribed in Vermont folk medicine are but different ways of presenting the body with potassium. Green leaves, plant and tree buds, tree barks, plant roots, fruits of the grape vine, cranberry bush (whereas cranberries grow in bogs on Cape Cod, in Vermont they grow on bushes) and apple tree all are sources of potassium.

In humans and animals alike, the body definitely wants potassium and if necessary will go to great lengths to get it. Take children for an example. It does not always please mothers when children eat dirt, but perhaps that is because they do not realize that instinctively children find the potassium needed for their bodily growth in the dirt.

A horse will chew the wood of his stall because the wood contains potassium. Put a section of tree limb in the manger for him to chew on, and he will stop chewing his stall. Calves will not chew the wood of their pens if apple cider vinegar is added to their drinking water. If cows are fed ocean kelp they will leave off licking their iron stanchions.

In the course of my interest in potassium as a means to winning the contest between bacteria and body cells, I applied potassium associated with other minerals to the soil in my flower garden. I had used potassium each year but then it occurred to me that what I was using lacked the associated minerals found with potassium in Nature.

Barre, Vermont, being the largest granite-cutting center in the world, I decided to try adding granite dust which, as it comes from the dust-removing device, is fine, like flour. Granite dust contains 5 per cent of potassium, and has associated with it sixteen minerals. When I applied it to the soil around my garden plants, a number of things happened.

Among my flowers, I have 125 plants of delphinium. Each year I had been having to combat a tiny mite which caused the leaves to curl up and turn black. These harmful mites were so small that I had to use a magnifying glass in order to see them crawling on the leaves. I used a spray but it did not do away with them. When I added the granite dust to the soil around the plants, these harmful mites deserted my garden and have not returned.

It has not been necessary to spray my collection of 60 rose bushes since I began applying the granite dust to them in the spring, midsummer, and fall. I have come to the conclusion that potassium alone is not as effective in producing results as potassium with associated minerals, some of which must activate the potassium.

Vermont folk medicine holds potassium to be the most important mineral, in fact the key mineral in the constellation of minerals. It is so essential to the life of every living thing that without it there would be no life. Nature has flung it about with such prodigality that one may say it is among the most generously and widely distributed of all the tissue minerals. Yet, notwithstanding its diffusion over the whole earth, the mineral potassium never occurs in a free state. It is never found pure, but always in combination with an acid.

Here in Vermont the topsoil is poor in potassium. Minerals in the soil hitchhike in the vegetation grown on the soil, in order to gain entrance to the body in animals and human beings eating land-grown foods. When one or more minerals are lacking in the soil, they are lacking in the food grown in that soil. When mineral-deficient food is eaten, the cells of the body are cheated of needed minerals on which they depend for balanced cell action. A disturbance in the physiology and body chemistry may follow, in due time producing symptoms of the presence of a clinical condition.

In the garden potassium is necessary to the production of the substances which give rigidity to the plant stems and increase their resistance to disease. Potassium is the power which changes seed into flower by progressive development. If potassium is lacking, the plant stops its evolution at some intermediate stage. The first tell-tale sign of potassium deficiency in a plant is cessation of growth for no discernible external reason. If the deficiency is not corrected, the plant slowly yellows and dies. Similarly in the human or animal body, when we note the presence of abnormal growth or failure to replace wornout tissues, we at once suspect an absence in the body of a sufficient amount of potassium to perform the appointed regulating function.

Potassium requirements are at a maximum when they are being used in infancy to build body tissues. But the requirements continue throughout life and there is no substitute for potassium.

The minerals that normally should be present in the daily food intake are necessary to the assimilation of food by the protoplasm in plants, animals, and humans. Protoplasm is the vitalizing, growth-controlling, health-sustaining, life-maintaining material not only of the plant cell but of the animal and human cells. When potassium is removed in the processing of foods, Nature's plans are interfered with. I am constantly being counseled by native Vermonters who live close to the soil to eat as little food as possible that comes out of a factory. Especially packaged cereals, they warn me, will lessen my ability to carry on sustained work.

Because potassium is associated with growth, I turned to the U.S. Draft Maps for the decade 1920–1930, to learn whether a lack of potassium in the Vermont topsoil would show up in them. In studying them I learned that Vermonters are underheight. I drew the conclusion that this lack of normal height was undoubtedly the result of the Vermont environment, with its characteristic lack in the topsoil of potassium.

If potassium lack produced this lack of height in human individuals the question arose as to whether it was also found in animals. From an issue of *Hoard's Dairyman,* which has a large circulation among Vermont farmers, I cut out a table which showed the normal height of different breeds of calves at birth, and as growth took place. With this table at hand I measured the height of 25 Jersey calves in a registered herd numbering 45. Of the 25 I measured, 17 were underheight. I then measured Jersey calves in two prize-winning Jersey herds; again, at birth, and as growth developed from month to month, the majority of calves were underheight.

This led me to another question. If potassium is responsible for normal growth, would a calf show normal height at birth if the mother were given potassium during her pregnancy?

In endeavoring to get the answer to this question, potassium was presented to the mother cow in four different ways:

1. Two ounces of apple cider vinegar was poured over each feeding twice a day.

2. Kelp from the ocean was added to the ration at each feeding, in the form of a cattle-food supplement marketed under the trade name of "Manamar."

3. The mother cow was given two onces of apple cider vinegar and three drops of Lugol's solution of iodine mixed together.

This was started at the beginning of the sixth month of the cow's pregnancy, poured over the ration at one feeding a day, three times a week. At the beginning of the last two weeks of pregnancy, two ounces of apple cider vinegar and three drops of Lugol's solution of iodine, mixed together, were poured over the ration at each feeding, twice a day.

4. The land was fertilized with potassium so that the hay, corn and other roughage grown would have a maximum potassium content.

These four methods all produced strong, rugged calves with a heavy coat of hair. They were normal in height at birth and were on their feet within five minutes of birth, nursing at the mother's udder within one half hour.

Along the same line, the potassium intake of mother goats was increased. This resulted in goat kids being larger at birth, up on their feet within 15 minutes after birth, hoofs hardened in 12 to 18 hours.

When apple cider vinegar was added to the drinking water of chickens, they feathered out quicker, grew tail feathers sooner and showed increased growth.

From the above variety of work it seemed reasonable to assume that here in Vermont our underheight is due to the lack of potassium in our topsoil and the removal of potassium in processing foods for market.

When underheight occurs it emphasizes the need of paying attention to the potassium intake during the period of growth. Controlled growth within the body, control of the processes within the body associated with normal growth, and normal replacement of worn-out body tissues depend on an adequate daily intake of potassium. When we note the presence of uncontrolled growth, such as the tendency to callous formation on the soles of the feet, or the failure to replace worn-out tissues as observed in loss of hair, decayed teeth, and fingernails that bend and tear, we must at once suspect the absence in the body of a sufficient amount of potassium to perform the regulating function of controlled growth.

I was very much interested in how native Vermonters living close to the soil check the rate of their own body growth, to learn whether it is as it should be. Somehow they had learned that it requires five months to grow a new thumbnail and ten months to grow a new nail for the big toe. With a file a mark is made at the base of the thumbnail, and at the base of the big toenail. The date when these marks were made is written down and kept handy for reference. At the end of five months, if growth is normal, this file mark on the thumbnail should be at its top, and at ten months the file mark on the big toenail should be at the outer end of the nail. If the file mark reaches either point before or after the expected date, it shows whether the growth rate in his body is more rapid or less rapid than normal. If less rapid it indicates the need of increasing the intake of potassium-rich foods, to speed up the rate of growth.

Potassium is to the soft tissues what calcium is to the hard tissues of the body. There is little doubt that potassium slows up the hardening processes that menace the whole blood-vessel system. Because the potassium present in apple cider vinegar makes the meat of the dairy cow or bull tender when it is slaughtered for beef, there is very little doubt that one of the functions of potassium is to keep the tissue soft and pliable.

Serious study of Vermont folk medicine leads to the matter of the taking in and giving out of fluid by the body cells. The taking in is referred to as hydration, the giving out as dehydration. Vermont folk medicine holds that bacteria needing moisture with which to maintain themselves get it by taking moisture from the body cells. But if there is enough potassium in each body cell it will draw moisture from the bacteria, instead of the bacteria taking moisture from the body cells. The constant contest between bacteria and body cells, therefore, determines whether the cell's attraction for water is strong enough to take it from the bacteria, or whether the moisture-attracting ability of the bacteria is strong enough to withdraw moisture from the body cells. It is by taking care to eat foods which are a source of potassium, such as fruit, berries, edible leaves, edible roots, and honey, and by the use of apple cider vinegar, that the body cells are provided with the moisture-attracting potassium needed to win the contest with bacteria. When the body cells seem to be losing the contest one can, by prescribing suitable treatment, turn the tide, making it impossible for the bacteria to win. The principle of the various modern drugs commonly used by organized medicine in the treatment of disease would appear to be powerful hydrating drugs, which enable the body cells to quickly take up fluid at the expense of the bacteria present, with the result that bacteria die and sickness is terminated.

One reason for the versatility of apple cider vinegar as a remedy in Vermont folk medicine is that it associates minerals with potassium. These are phosphorus, chlorine, sodium, magnesium, calcium, sulfur, iron, fluorine, silicon, and many trace minerals.

As an example of the eagerness of animals to get the potassium and associated minerals derived from the apple, the following furnished experimental evidence. A barrel which had held apple cider vinegar needed a thorough washing to remove the accumulated mother-of-vinegar, the stringy, sticky, bacterial residue, before being refilled with fresh apple juice from the cider mill to be aged into apple cider vinegar.

The barrel was taken to a pasture where a dairy herd was at the time. As soon as the water in which the barrel was washed was emptied out onto the ground, the cows fought one another to get at the wetness. Not only did they eat all the grass, but they ate the dirt underneath, which had been soaked with the barrel washings.

"An apple a day keeps the doctor away" is a familiar adage. Its kernel of truth is that apples are very healthful for the human system. Apple cider vinegar carries all the above-named minerals over from the original apple. Whether used in the form of apple juice, apple cider, or apple cider vinegar, treatment results are the same because each is a source of these minerals. If you experiment with different vinegars you will learn that no others will produce the same treatment results as apple cider vinegar. Wine vinegar, used by the Italians, comes nearest to the effects of apple cider vinegar. For medicinal purposes the apple cider vinegar should be made from the crushed whole apples. There are on the market vinegars which are made from apple peelings and cores after the apple pulp has been used for some other commercial purpose. However, the label will state whether an apple cider vinegar is made of the whole apple. Such brands as Sterling and Heinz are suitable for medicinal use because they are made from whole apples.

Following the line of changes when the whole apple is crushed to make apple cider vinegar, it is found that the healthful properties in the original apple are passed down to the apple cider vinegar, the only change being that the sugars of the fruit are rendered into the acid which is vinegar. It is helpful to know precisely what vinegar does in your digestive tract, and how and why two teaspoonfuls of apple cider vinegar to a glass of water at each meal is helpful in maintaining the health of your digestive tract and, in turn, the all-around health of your body.

I may give this illustration, which I hope will not unduly disconcert the reader. To observe what happens to bacterial life when vinegar is used, get an angleworm from the garden and put it on a board or other hard surface where you may observe it. Now pour apple cider vinegar over it. First, it writhes as though in pain. In a few seconds it becomes motionless. In a few seconds more its pink color disappears and it turns white. The vinegar has caused loss of life in just those few seconds, for the worm is now dead. In the same way apple cider vinegar will destroy bacteria in your digestive tract.

Let me present four cases which will illustrate what I have written.

Two sisters planned to have fish for dinner. After smelling the fish, one of them said she believed it was spoiled and should be thrown away. The other sister smelled it too, and believed it was all right. So the fish was cooked and served.

I had happened to teach one of the sisters to add two teaspoonfuls of apple cider vinegar to a glass of water whenever she suspected that some food which was taken was not quite right. She was a cooking-school graduate and from time to time we discussed the preparation of foods for eating.

So the first thing she did now before starting to eat the fish was to put two teaspoonfuls of apple cider vinegar in a glass of water and take two or three swallows before eating. She suggested that her sister, whom she was visiting in Massachusetts, do likewise, but the sister thought it unnecessary. In a short time the Massachusetts sister developed an attack of diarrhea whereas her Vermont sister, having protected herself by the dose of apple cider vinegar and water, maintained a normal digestive tract and suffered no discomfort.

A young couple accepted an invitation to a weenie roast. As I had taught the wife, she took some apple cider vinegar in a glass of water before leaving home; she wanted her husband to do the same but he was sure it was not necessary. When they came home the wife took another glass of the vinegar and water and was perfectly comfortable. The husband, however, developed a sharp attack of diarrhea with vomiting.

At a Shriners summer outing here in Vermont, lobster salad was served at dinner. Unfortunately the salad was spoiled and nineteen Barre people developed severe diarrhea, complicated in some cases by vomiting. One of the diners had taken precautions. As I had advised him when there was any chance that food might have become spoiled, he had brought along a little bottle of apple cider vinegar to the affair. At the outset of dinner he poured a liberal amount into his glass of water. It happened that he was particularly fond of lobster salad and he had two extra helpings. Whereas many of his table companions suffered bad effects from the spoiled lobster, the apple cider vinegar had so sterilized it in his digestive tract that nothing disagreeable happened to him.

At another time, when I was attending a national medical meeting, a bellboy tapped me on the shoulder, asking me to call the number of a certain room. One of my medical colleagues answered and asked me to come up immediately, as he was sick and needed help.

He had awakened in the night feeling his digestive tract off balance. He had diarrhea and there was vomiting. It was now ten o'clock in the morning. I fetched from my room the bottle of apple cider vinegar which I always carry when on a trip away from home. Putting one teaspoonful of the vinegar in a glass of water, I gave him a teaspoonful of the mixture every five minutes. When there is food poisoning with vomiting, if you should attempt to drink a whole glass at once, the stomach would not accept it. But the small amount every few minutes can be kept down. An ordinary drinking glass will hold about fifty teaspoonfuls, and teaspoonful doses will require about four hours. When the contents of the first glassful have been taken, another should be prepared in the same way and the dose increased to two teaspoonfuls every five minutes. This will add about two hours more of treatment. A third glassful should be prepared and taken one small swallow every fifteen minutes.

If you awaken in the morning with diarrhea and vomiting you should be able to straighten out your stomach and bowel condition by following this apple cider vinegar and water treatment through the day. By suppertime you should be able to eat a small meal of easily digested food. For two or three days you should take a glass of the mixture at each meal, to continue the stomach and bowels in good health. My medical friend, having followed the above-outlined schedule, was able to eat his supper.

Incidentally, I think the cases well illustrate the utter simplicity, convenience, and completeness in themselves of many treatments used in Vermont folk medicine. In former times, before one could telephone for the doctor, people necessarily acquainted themselves with ways to use Nature's leaves, herbs, and fruits to relieve sickness and restore body balance. Every pantry can easily contain apple cider vinegar, and a small bottle is as easy to take along in luggage as a tube of toothpaste.

In speaking of the dosage taken by my medical friend to clear up his difficulty, I touched on a point which has been the subject of much experimentation by Vermont folk medicine during the passing years. In trying to learn the correct medicinal dose, I found that it was an individual matter. Some people have found that the dose for them was one teaspoonful of the apple cider vinegar to a glass of water. Others say they pour the vinegar into an ordinary glass to the measure of the width of one finger, then filling the glass with water. Still others reported, variously, that two fingers and three fingers of vinegar in the glass of water were correct. I have also come across those who made the mixture half-and-half. And I also found one woman, in the early forties, who craved the sour from time to time and would drink a glass of apple cider vinegar neat, as the saying goes. I asked her what happened when she did this. Nothing, she said, except that she did not crave the sour any more for a time.

If for any reason apple cider vinegar is not accepted by the body, try taking a small glass of apple juice, sometimes called sweet cider, so that the body may receive the healthful properties of the apple.

Having observed what apple cider vinegar does to improve the health of the digestive tract, let us observe its effect on the kidneys and bladder.

When the human individual taking two teaspoonfuls of the vinegar in a glass of water each meal passes urine in a vessel at night, the following morning it will be noted that no red dustlike deposit is present in the vessel; this shows that a marked chemical change has taken place in the urine.

If there is inflammation in the kidney called pyelitis, in which pus cells are present in the urine, generally the condition will be cleared up by taking a mixture of two teaspoonfuls of apple cider vinegar in a glass of water.

For fifteen years a married woman forty-eight years of age had been subject to attacks of pyelitis. Attacks came sometimes as often as every six weeks, and never was she free of them for more than two or three months. She began taking apple cider vinegar and found she was free from pyelitis. When she had been free of any attack for one year she discounted the apple cider vinegar, believing she no longer needed it. Four weeks later the pyelitis developed again, with chills, a temperature of 103 degrees, and pain in the region of the left kidney. She returned to taking the apple cider vinegar and the clinical condition quieted down.

We hear a great deal these days of the effects on daily living of such disturbances as chronic fatigue, chronic headache, including the perplexing migraine type, high blood pressure, dizziness, and, especially because of its association with heart trouble, of overweight. Potassium and associated minerals play a very important part in the approaches of Vermont folk medicine to treatment of these difficulties and I should like to go into some observations made in the course of my studies.

OVERWEIGHT

Among Vermonters a statement is in common use to the effect that "You can reduce by the tape measure, but you cannot reduce by the scales." They call attention by this statement to the fact that changes in the bony framework of the body, and changes in the body tissues such as the muscles, can offset the loss of fat. When the weight of the individual increases above normal, it well may be due to an excessive amount of storage tissue deposited as fat.

There are different ways of estimating what one's weight should be. Vermont folk medicine estimates it this way: Twice around the wrist equals once around the lower part of the neck. Twice around the neck at its lowest part equals once around the waist.

A good rule for deciding what your own weight should be, devised by Dr. Lulu Hunt Peters, is as follows:

1. Measure your height without your shoes.
2. Take the number of inches over 5 feet and multiply this by 5½.
3. To this number add 110. This will give you your ideal weight.

For example, suppose your height without shoes is 5 feet 7 inches. Take the seven inches and multiply it by 5½, which makes 38½. Now add 110. The answer is 148½, which is the ideal weight.

If you are under 5 feet, then multiply the number of inches under 5 feet by 5½ and subtract the answer from 110.

If the waist measurement is greater than that of the chest, or the chin is inclined to be double, then it is generally safe to conclude that the normal physiology and biochemistry in the body are disturbed. When this happens Vermont folk medicine depends on apple cider vinegar to bring about a disappearance of excess fat.

If a woman whose dress fits tightly will sip two teaspoonfuls of apple cider vinegar in a glass of water at each meal, generally she will find at the end of two months that she can take her dress in one inch at the waistline. At the end of two more months she will be able to take it in another inch, and by the end of the fifth month one more inch. At the end of one year of taking apple cider vinegar in this amount a woman who has taken a size 50 dress will be able to take a size 42, and one who has taken a size 20, to take a size 18. At the end of the same time a younger woman who has worn a size 16 will be able to take a size 14.

The loss of weight will be gradual. If a woman between 5 feet and 5 feet 6 inches tall weighing 210 pounds takes two teaspoonfuls of apple cider vinegar in a glass of water at each meal, she will weigh about 180 pounds at the end of two years. If a man has a paunch, he will lose the paunch in two years' time. The apple cider vinegar will have made it possible to burn the fat in the body instead of storing it, increasing the body weight.

No change in the daily food intake is made except to avoid foods that experience has shown the individual will increase the amount of fat deposited in the body.

If continued day after day, this treatment for excess weight is completely simple, and completely effective. If the daily routine happens to be such that it is not practical to take it at each meal, a dose can be taken in the morning, another at bedtime, with the third taken at some convenient time in between.

CHRONIC FATIGUE

Whether we wish to or not, you and I must follow some sort of health pathway our whole life long. We must have good health to accomplish whatever represents our goal in our social, professional, or business life. To live successfully one must live long enough to accomplish what one dreamed of doing, and be healthy while doing so. We must condition ourselves to the work we do.

Without long life and accompanying good health no average human being can live to the hilt. To be obliged to drop anchor because of frequent sickness or continued poor health, having to watch the rest of the world pass by, is to be cheated out of some of life. To be out of the running because of a physical breakdown when one is at or nearing the peak of social, business, and professional life is disastrously disappointing. Rightly, life should not be marked with unfulfilled beginnings or with brilliant promise never brought to fruition because time must be spent in regaining health. During apprenticeship days professional, business, and social abilities must be free to ripen, and the abilities mature at a point in life when there is still enough of life to reap and enjoy the rewards.

As a rule your body has a warning period, which you should heed, before succumbing to the ravages of illness. As an alarm clock wakes you from sound sleep, these warnings are a bodily alarm reaction which should be sufficient to awaken you to the need of checking your daily routine, to learn whether, and where, you are out of step with those laws of Nature which were devised for the human machine.

Chronic fatigue is one such warning. Suddenly, perhaps, you find that you are easily fatigued. A night's rest does not remove this sense of fatigue and you are exhausted when you rise in the morning. The day's work ceases to give you any pleasure. You give up one outside activity after another. You have lost your drive and initiative and have spells of deep discouragement. You may have real mental ability, and know you have it in you to do very much better than you are doing—if only you could get rid of this ever-present tired feeling! If you could only match your mental ability with the proper physical ability, you could go ahead rapidly in your chosen work. Occasionally you do have a good day, when you feel equal to anything and everything the day demands. While it lasts, you accomplish much. You wonder why you can't feel this way all the time.

If you have chronic fatigue, let us first check up on the amount of time you sleep at night. When do you go to bed? When do you get up in the morning?

Remember that artificial lighting after sundown was invented by man. The present modern timetable of daily activities aided by artificial lighting is not the timetable set by Nature. Nature's timetable of lighting begins at sunrise and ends with sunset. Though it is impractical for most of us, who need to live in relation to the modern tempo around us, to begin our work at sunrise and end it at sunset, we must nevertheless balance work and rest as nearly as possible in keeping with Nature's wise plan. One essential is to get as many hours in bed before midnight as you can. We know of individuals, of course, who require only a few hours of sleep to bring them fresh to the beginning of the new day. But we are not among them if we have developed chronic fatigue, with loss of "the will to win."

Quite possibly you may find it difficult to fall asleep at night, and to sleep soundly after you are asleep. If this is true you should become interested in honey. Acting as a sedative to the body, honey is the best remedy of all to produce sleep. Being a predigested sugar, digested in the stomach of the honey bee, honey requires no digestion by the human stomach but is ready to be used immediately by the body. Twenty minutes after it is taken by mouth, it is in the blood stream. To cope with chronic fatigue Vermont folk medicine knows no better treatment than this: add three teaspoonfuls of apple cider vinegar to a cup of honey, placing the mixture in a wide-mouthed bottle or jar that will admit a teaspoon, and keep the jar in the bedroom. Take two teaspoonfuls of the mixture when preparing for bed. They will enable you to fall asleep within a half hour after getting into bed. If by the end of an hour you should not be asleep, take two teaspoonfuls more of the mixture. In cases of extreme wakefulness, it may take several such doses, and if you should awake during the night and feel unable to get back to sleep you should take still another. This is far superior to the usual "lullaby pills" because it is a treatment based on Nature's own infallible knowledge of bodily requirements; being harmless, it can be taken indefinitely. The honey may be taken by itself to produce sleep, but Vermont folk medicine teaches that the combining of it with the apple cider vinegar is more effective.

On rising in the morning the reaction of the urine should be tested with Squibb's Nitrazine Paper. A normal urine reaction is acid; the paper should turn yellow. This taking of the reaction in the morning will enable you to know whether your night's rest has been sufficient to restore your body chemistry to normal. This in turn enables you to estimate how much reserve energy you have available on deposit in your body for your day's work. As reserve energy is deposited in your body by hours of body rest, sleep, freedom from worry, and an avoidance of foods that produce an alkaline urine reaction, your morning urine reaction, shown by the Squibb's Nitrazine Paper, will tell you if you have overdrawn your reserve energy account and need to make a deposit by more body rest and sleep, less worry, and more careful attention to daily food intake, avoiding foods producing an alkaline urine reaction.

If you are subject to chronic fatigue you must learn by constant practice to rest wherever you are at the moment. I think it was a former president of Dartmouth College who made famous a dictum, "I never stand if I can sit; I never run if I can walk; I never sit up if I can lie down." Though most of us would perhaps find it difficult to govern our lives by this, it does imply a method of avoiding tension through sitting, walking, or relaxing in order to economize the expenditure of reserve energy.

If the morning urine reaction indicates that the amount of reserve energy on deposit is very low, then it would be wise to take a hand bath of apple cider vinegar and water. To a half glass of warm water add one teaspoonful of apple cider vinegar. Cup the palm of the hand and pour into it from the glass about one teaspoonful of the solution. First apply the solution to one arm and shoulder. Then apply another teaspoonful of the solution to the opposite arm and shoulder. In succession apply equal amounts to the chest, stomach, back, the upper half of each leg, the lower half, finally to each foot. Do not use a towel. Instead, rub the skin surface of the body with both hands until it has completely taken up the solution, which it will do very quickly.

It will surprise some people if I say that, in getting rid of your chronic fatigue, you must seriously consider ceasing to use soap. Test the moistened surface of a cake of soap with a strip of the Squibb's Nitrazine Paper and you will observe that the paper turns a dark blue, indicating that it is very alkaline in reaction. Being alkaline, soap helps to create in your body the very chronic fatigue you wish to get rid of. After all, soap is man-made; you do not find it growing on trees or bushes. On the other hand, Nature has spread acid about generously, and you find it growing in many forms on plants.

If the cleansing agent you use on your skin is acid, you present the skin with the element which is normal to it, namely acid. When the skin is acid it appears to attract blood to it, whereas when an alkaline solution is applied, such as is represented by soap and water, the skin is apt to be pale and make-up may have to be used to give the appearance of health. The presence of the normal amount of blood in the skin gives it a pink glow; conversely, a pale skin generally indicates a starving for acid. If it is necessary to use soap to remove dirt, as little as possible should be used, and you should follow using it by an application of apple cider vinegar and water solution, in order to leave the skin normally acid in reaction.

The same rule applies to the tub bath. Instead of using soap, add a half pint of apple cider vinegar to the water and remain in the water for at least fifteen minutes so that the skin surface of the body may have a chance to absorb some of the acid water. With the tub bath too, if you must use soap, use as little as possible and be sure to leave the skin acid by an application of the apple cider vinegar and water solution.

You may say, "But how shall I know that my skin is not acid in reaction?" There will be a very simple sign. The skin which is alkaline in reaction will itch. An itching of your head or the skin surface of your body is the body's way of telling you to stop using soap and start using a cleansing agent which will stop the itching by returning the skin to its normal acid reaction. If you are a man, and your scalp itches, add one teaspoonful of apple cider vinegar to a glass of water, dip the comb in the solution and comb the hair. Continue until the hair is quite saturated. A woman has a bit more of a problem. If her hair has a permanent wave, and she combs the apple cider vinegar and water solution into it, it will straighten out the permanent. She will probably choose, therefore, to treat the scalp at about the time she is going to have a shampoo anyway.

Having taken the skin into account in relation to chronic fatigue, let us think about the food intake with which we build and rebuild the body. There are several foods you should avoid eating if you have a problem of chronic fatigue. Here we may borrow guidance from the animals. For instance, birds will not eat wheat. If a prepared bird food containing wheat is put out for them, they will separate out the wheat and eat the rest. Farmers in Vermont tell me that if wheat is mixed in with scratch feed hens will not eat it at all or, if very hungry, will only eat it last. If there is too much wheat in a cow's ration she will not eat it. Animals seem to know instinctively that eating is for strength, not to produce weariness and weakness, and that if they eat wheat they will produce weak offspring.

The person who suffers from chronic fatigue should learn to live out of the ocean because one reason for the fatigue is a need for more iodine and other minerals abundantly present in fish and other ocean food. Baked beans too are generally well accepted by the body of one troubled with chronic fatigue; when they are they may be taken as many as three times during the week. In Vermont it is a food custom to serve them with vinegar. Some people like to put vinegar directly on the beans but others prefer to get the vinegar in a proportion of one teaspoonful to a glass of water, sipped a swallow or two at a time during the meal. All in all, each individual with chronic fatigue should, by carrying on some research and experimentation, be able in time to determine just what foods produce for them the wanted acid reaction and what foods to avoid because they will produce the unwanted alkaline reaction.

CHRONIC HEADACHE

Chronic headaches are blamed on the eyes, the stomach, the kidneys, the liver, and the sinuses.

There are several types of chronic headache. Some are associated with organic disease, such as kidney disease. Some are known as *psychogenic,* or tension, headaches. For these the emotions—hate, fear, anxiety—are given the blame. Most annoying of all to the individual is the migraine headache.

Migraine headaches are inherited and affect people of a definite physical type. They occur in people having considerable energy and good intelligence. These people are sensitive and sympathetic. They are also fussy, demanding, aggressive, and ambitious. I have heard migraine headaches called "the price man pays for his ambitions."

There is a tendency, even among doctors, to classify most baffling types of chronic headaches as migraine. The real, or classic, symptoms, however, are pretty specific. The victim has an "aura" or pre-headache warning even before it starts. There are spots or flashes of light before the eyes. The ache is on one side of the head—the word *migraine* means "half a head"—and there is often nausea or other digestive disturbances.

Emotions, fears, and anxieties trigger the migraine-headache process. As the individual grows older, attacks diminish. It is unusual to have migraine headache after sixty years of age. This is probably partly because an individual grows calmer and better adjusted to circumstances as he grows older.

I have spent a great deal of time studying migraine headaches with the cooperation of individuals suffering them who were willing to serve as human guinea pigs. As with so many other conditions indicating that the body was off balance, the first step was to learn whether migraine headaches appeared on an alkaline or an acid urine reaction, as shown by the Squibb's Nitrazine Paper method previously described. When the urine reaction is shifted to acid, migraine headaches were less frequent, much less severe if they did come, or disappeared altogether. Obviously the salvation of the person who suffers from them lies in understanding the various factors which will produce the alkaline reaction, and then controlling and combating them.

The daily intake of acid should be increased by the apple cider vinegar method, which is easy and positive. Too, many migraine headaches are prevented by the use of honey. Two teaspoonfuls of honey taken at each meal may well prevent an attack. If the headache has appeared, however, take a tablespoonful of honey at once. Since it requires no process of digestion and will quickly be in the blood stream, the headache often will begin to lessen by the end of a half hour. If not, another tablespoonful of honey should be taken. Its sedative effect on the body is just what is needed by the characteristics which produce this type of headache.

Vermont folk medicine finds another application of apple cider vinegar efficacious in treating migraine headaches. It is a vaporizing method. Put equal parts of the vinegar and water in a small basin on the stove, allowing it to boil slowly.

When fumes begin to rise from the basin, lean the head over it until the fumes are comfortably strong. Inhale them for 75 breaths. Generally you will find that the headache stops for about a half hour. If it starts again it will be about 50 per cent less severe. The use of headache tablets can be stopped if the apple cider vinegar fumes method is employed.

HIGH BLOOD PRESSURE

Few problems are of more importance than the treatment of high blood pressure. It is both a common and a serious condition. There is almost certainly a relationship between increased blood pressure and an individual's adjustment to his environment.

When the demands of environment are not beyond his capacity to meet them, the individual lives a strenuous, successful life with the usual life expectancy. When the demands seem excessive, however, and the individual does not know how to adapt himself to them, his body mechanism falls out of balance; as it does so, sustained high blood pressure may be one of the manifest signs.

High blood pressure as a problem of health is growing in importance, since it is an associated factor in three fourths of the yearly deaths due to heart and kidney disease. Whether high blood pressure is a disease or a symptom is a much-debated question. When we know the cause of the clinical condition, we look upon the associated high blood pressure as a symptom; when we do not know the cause we look on the high blood pressure as the disease itself.

Individuals with high blood pressure are usually divided into two groups. When its cause cannot be attributed to a known disease the term *essential hypertension* is employed. The condition is often referred to as *primary high blood pressure*. When a demonstrated cause can be observed, the term *secondary high blood pressure* is used.

From medical literature on the subject the mechanism

seems clear by which blood pressure is elevated to essential hypertension. Throughout the body an increased resistance is offered to the flow of blood through the small blood vessels called arterioles. In the early stages of hypertension the constriction of these arterioles is easily reversible and during sleep the blood pressure returns to normal, indicating relaxation of the arterioles.

However, in most cases this reversibility is lost as time passes, and rest will not cause the blood pressure to return to normal. According to organized medicine arteriolar constriction in high blood pressure appears to have two main explanations. One attributes the state to overactivity of the sympathetic nervous system, which organizes the body for fight or flight and causes widespread constriction of the arterioles. The second explanation is that chemical substances circulate in the blood and produce a narrowing of the arterioles.

Continued contact with patients showing high blood pressure suggests that in most of them a strong personality factor is presented. The majority of patients having essential hypertension are dynamic, hard-driving, non-procrastinating, with the desire and ability to accomplish much in a short space of time. This is the race-horse type of individual. Careful questioning of the individual and his relatives generally reveals that this personality has not developed after the high blood pressure but represents natural tendencies seen in the individual as far back as can be remembered.

When individuals with high blood pressure are studied from week to week, on the basis of being seen one or more times a week for one or more years, a number of things about high blood pressure will be learned. It will be observed, for example, that it is not a fixed physiologic constant but varies from day to day and week to week. The variation occurs with physical activity, rest, ingestion of foods, weather, pain, nervous stress and strain. Especially are weather changes an influence. Blood pressure is highest in cold weather, lowest in warm. Here in Vermont it is highest during January and February, lowest in July and August. The first few readings taken in a doctor's office are very apt to be close to the maximum pressure because of apprehension in the individual, and his natural tension during a physical examination. Such readings are not necessarily representative of the individual's blood pressure level under ordinary circumstances. As individual and examiner become better acquainted the individual is no longer affected by this initial tension.

When high blood pressure is present, what attitude does Vermont folk medicine take?

Nature's arranged plan for man provides for a food intake, represented by fruits, berries, edible leaves, and honey, that is rich in carbohydrates rather than a food intake, represented by eggs, meat, milk, cheese, peas, beans, and nuts, that is rich in proteins. Man takes his first step toward high blood pressure when he changes this plan to a low carbohydrate-high protein daily food intake. He makes this change to increased protein intake in order to create within his body the needed energy to meet the more exacting needs of an increased tempo of living. We find this organizing of the body illustrated, for example, when African tribes kill and eat a cow before starting on a lion hunt for the purpose of getting rid of lions which prey on livestock and members of the tribe. By eating the protein represented by the meat they have better organized their bodies for the aggressive action constituting the hunt.

Now an increased daily intake of protein would not be harmful if the increased alkalinity of the blood it produced was offset by a corresponding increase of acid in organic form, such as apple cider vinegar, apples, grapes, cranberries, or their juices. The blood is always alkaline in reaction. But this alkalinity may be increased or decreased. If alkalinity is increased, the blood thickens and precipitates its solids in tiny flakes. The walls of the tiny blood vessels in the arterial tree allow the fluid part of the blood to pass through similar in manner to the way ink will pass through blotting paper. But thickened blood will not pass through the blotting-paper-like walls of the tiny blood vessels as easily as it should. The little flakes plug some of the tiny blood vessels and after a time there is a backing-up of the blood, with a resulting increase in blood pressure.

What does Vermont folk medicine say to do about this?

1. Increase the daily intake of acid in organic form. This may be in the form of apples, grapes, cranberries or their juices. Each day you would need to take the equivalent of four glasses of juice. This may be with or without meals, at the time most convenient for you. If you use apple cider vinegar as the source of acid, take two teaspoonfuls in a glass of water.

2. You should review your daily food intake and determine the comparison between its protein and carbohydrate content. If the protein is higher, try to better balance the two.

3. Exchange wheat foods for corn. As the kidneys are spill-over organs, the alkaline urine reaction produced by wheat foods, refined sugar, and meat is a sign that the blood wishes to reduce its alkaline content.

4. Common table salt attracts and holds fluid in the body; hence salty foods should be given up by those having high blood pressure. Any individual is familiar with the desire to drink water after taking salty foods. Part of the additional fluid demanded by the salt is held in the blood stream until it can be eliminated from the body, and this holding of excess fluid in the blood stream produces a rise in blood pressure. If salt and salty foods are given up the blood will readily give up the excess fluid and the blood pressure will drop to the extent for which the salt intake was responsible.

The effect of honey is quite opposite. Honey is a magnet for water. If it is taken at each meal it draws excess fluid from the blood, lowering blood pressure and, being helpfully sedative, alleviating any tension disturbing the nervous system.

A Vermont woman showed an unusually high blood pressure reading of nearly 300 when it was taken at a nationally known clinic. The staff was surprised that she was even alive. However, by controlling the alkalinity of her blood in the manner taught by Vermont folk medicine, she was able to live to the age of eighty-four years. I took the blood pressure of her daughter, when the daughter was in her early fifties Her blood pressure was a high 225. By following the course established for her mother, she lived to be eighty-one years old.

DIZZINESS

Because Vermont folk medicine is successful in treating dizziness, I spent some time studying the problem and the treatment. As I went along I noted that Vermont might reasonably be described as the land of dizziness, for it is a common symptom.

A continued study over many years brings to light four types of dizziness:

Type 1. Momentary dizziness. The individual does not like high places and is very apt to cling to the stair railing while going downstairs, especially when in public buildings. He finds it difficult to look down from a height. Coordination between feet and head does not seem to be good and when going downstairs he must look at each step as he goes along.

Type 2. This is associated with change of position of the body. If one gets up suddenly, he is obliged to grasp some object to keep from falling. Glasses are often worn with the hope that they will diminish the dizziness. On awakening in the morning, this type of sufferer finds it necessary to sit on the edge of the bed for from five to fifteen minutes before he can walk across the room without dizziness. After he has been up for an hour or two the dizziness may have passed off. Type 2 individuals are often treated for biliousness with the idea that it is the cause of the dizziness.

Type 3. This individual is obliged to remain in bed days at a time because of a persistent dizziness, making it impossible to be up and dressed. He loses his sense of direction and may fall.

There does not seem to be any nausea connected with this type, nor do objects in the room go round.

Type 4. A Type 4 individual has attacks of severe dizziness accompanied by nausea, noises in the ears, and occasionally impaired hearing. Such an individual will be confined to bed for weeks at a time because of dizziness accompanied by rotation of objects in the room. He is unable to stand on his feet without falling down and, if he must walk, will need a person on either side to steady him.

The background of dizziness is an alkaline reaction of the urine. When the reaction is shifted to acid dizziness will be very much less, or disappears altogether. To prevent dizziness, Vermont folk medicine employs the apple cider vinegar treatment, with timing and dosage similar to applications to other difficulties. That an individual may suffer dizziness or be free from it depends on how willing he is to so order his life as to maintain an acid urine reaction.

A word of advice, however. Do not expect that, because you have taken apple cider vinegar one or two times today, you will be free of dizziness tomorrow and from then on. You should notice some lessening of the dizziness at the end of two weeks if you faithfully observe the folk-medicine rule for the apple cider vinegar dosage, and a further lessening by the end of one month.

SORE THROAT

The remedy most often used in Vermont folk medicine to treat sore throat is a gargle of apple cider vinegar. The mixture is one teaspoonful of the vinegar to a glass of water. One mouthful of the solution is gargled every hour, and swallowed after the gargling. This is followed by a second mouthful, used in the same manner.

As to the object of swallowing the gargle solution, the folk-medicine belief is that in this way it reaches all parts of the lower throat not reached by the gargling itself. As soreness in the throat lessens, intervals between gargling may be changed to once every two hours.

Much to my surprise I learned that this treatment could cure a streptococcic sore throat in 24 hours. As a rule the patient became free of symptoms before I got the report back from the Vermont state laboratory stating that the throat culture sent showed the presence of streptococci. Also I found that if a membrane was present on the tonsils, it disappeared in 12 hours' time.

RELATION OF POTASSIUM TO MUCUS

When walking week after week back and forth in front of dairy cow herds, studying the heads, and whether appetites were as they should be, I observed that some of the cows had watery eyes. At times tears ran down their faces, causing them to look as though they were crying. They were troubled too by wet noses, as shown by the way they ran the tongue up each nostril. Some cows also coughed, indicating an excess of mucus in the throat.

Medical literature having taught me that potassium is insatiably thirsty, being a magnet for water, the practice was started of pouring two ounces of apple cider vinegar over each cow's ration for the two feedings per day. Right away the wetness of eyes and nose and the coughing ceased. The only reasonable conclusion seemed that lack of sufficient potassium in the daily food intake had made it impossible for the cow's body to use the fluid. The eye, nose, and cough manifestations were the spontaneous effort to get rid of water in the body. Supplying the needed potassium through the ration brought about the process of dehydration. An excess of mucus was no longer present and the proportion of moisture to the body became normal.

When I see a patient, generally one who is elderly, who complains of wetness of the eyes, it is natural to adapt the approach learned from studying the dairy herd. A mixture is prepared of one teaspoonful of apple cider vinegar and one drop of Lugol's solution of iodine to a glass of water. The contents are stirred and taken in the course of one meal each day as one would take coffee or tea. This is to be continued for a period of two weeks.

At the end of that time a patient reported progress made in the drying up of the eyes. If necessary the treatment can be continued another two weeks; thereafter on Tuesday and Friday of each week, to prevent a return of the difficulty.

I have found the above treatment of value also in treating patients wishing "something done for a seepage from my sinuses." Generally, one or two weeks are required to stop a watery discharge from the nose. One must also make sure to ask the patient to discontinue citrus fruits and juices, for the reason that they alone may be responsible for a wet nose.

With a better understanding of potassium, it is not difficult to see its relation to postnasal drip, and its power, by attracting fluid and removing it from the body by way of the kidneys, to reduce postnasal drip naturally. If, in addition to the intake of potassium, the patient is reminded to omit foods made from wheat, replacing them with rye and cornmeal foods, and to avoid the citrus juices and fruits, many causes of postnasal drip will soon clear up.

"How can I tell the signs of a lack of potassium in the body?" you wonder.

1. There is some loss of mental alertness. Making decisions is a bit more difficult. The memory is not as efficient as it used to be.

2. Mental and muscle fatigue appear more often and more easily. You lack muscular endurance. You tire easily.

3. You note that you are more sensitive to cold. You prefer warm food to cold desserts. You are very apt to have cold hands and feet.

4. Calluses are very apt to appear on the bottoms of your feet. Corns build up easily.

5. You are very apt to be troubled by constipation.

6. You are more susceptible to sickness. It is very easy to catch cold.

7. At times there may be loss of appetite, and also at times nausea and vomiting.

8. Cuts and bruises heal slowly.

9. The skin of your body is very apt to itch.

10. You may have more tooth decay than it would seem you should.

11. Pimples may appear on your skin surface.

12. You are apt to have twitching of the eyelids, or the corner of your mouth.

13. You are apt to have cramps in the body muscles, especially the leg muscles. These are apt to occur during the night.

14. It is more difficult for you to relax.

15. You may have difficulty in sleeping well at night.

16. One or more joints of your body may develop soreness. It leads you to feel that arthritis may be developing.

The older you grow, the greater should be your daily intake of potassium. As a rule you should take into your body twice as much potassium, in the form of honey, fresh vegetables, fruits, and berries, as you do sodium, in the form of salty foods and table salt. Potassium is important not only for continued good health, because of the functions it performs in the body, but because of the delicate balance found between potassium and sodium in the body.

There are a number of easy ways whereby one may increase one's potassium intake:

1. Paprika is a rich source of potassium. It can be shaken on food once or twice a day.

2. We have frequently noted the mixture of apple cider vinegar and honey in a glass of water as another source.

3. A glass of grape juice twice a day, or of apple or cranberry juice, furnishes needed potassium in agreeable form.

As you experiment with different sources of potassium you

will probably learn that one influences you more than the others and you will want to use it more often than the others.

Grape juice is particularly acceptable to many individuals as a source of potassium. We are fortunate here in Vermont, for grapes grow wild here and native Vermonters have a long-standing habit of gathering wild grapes and making their own grape juice.

I spent some time in trying to learn more about grape juice.

The chemical composition and nourishment value of the edible portion of the grape, exclusive of skin and seeds, has been determined at the experiment stations of the U.S. Department of Agriculture and found to be as follows:

	Per cent
Water	77.4
Protein	1.3
Fat	1.6
Carbohydrates	19.2
Ash	0.5

Analysis of the mineral content of grape juice shows the following minerals per 100 grams:

	Per cent
Potassium	11.49
Sodium	0.97
Calcium	1.63
Magnesium	1.21
Iron	0.36
Phosphorus	7.08
Sulfur	1.01
Chlorine	0.42

Grape juice quenches thirst promptly, even when taken in small amounts. The rapid action of grape juice is due to the fact that grape sugar is taken immediately into the circulation without undergoing any process of digestion. On this account there is no undue tax on the organs of digestion and assimilation.

It is worthwhile to understand the relation of potassium to iron, to calcium, and to sodium.

When soil is potassium-poor, corn grown in the soil will rot in the roots and will also be covered by many and diverse fungi and molds. There will be a blocking of the nodes of joints by a reddish precipitate that shuts off the circulation of the sap from root to leaves, and leaves to roots. Conversely, when potassium is added to the soil, corn will grow tall, strong, and healthy; no longer do molds and fungi appear or ears and roots rot, nor do precipitated minerals block the sap channels at nodes and leaves.

When examining the blocked sap nodes, a few drops of dilute hydrochloric acid followed by a few drops of a solution of potassium ferrocyanide causes these nodes to turn red. This indicates that it is iron that had blocked the sap channels. Likewise, when the cut stalk ends are placed in a solution of methylene blue, the fact is disclosed that these channels were almost completely blocked by the iron deposits.

Let us leave the vegetable world, turning to animal, and human, bodies. We know that both have a similar lymph circulation, and that this lymph circulation has its channels, spaces, nodes, and glands. We know too, from contact with patients, that these glands block and swell. Also, by reason of blisters and bloating of tissues, we know that lymph is colorless, like tree sap, and that not only is it the nutrient of tissue life, but it also gives it oxygen and carries away the waste material resulting from the vital activity of the cells.

At once a number of questions come to mind. Cannot the lymph channels become blocked in the animal and human body, as described in diseased corn? Can iron become deposited in lymph spaces, lymph nodes, and various organs of the body? When a potassium deficiency is present in the animal and human bodies, can the body be invaded by fungi and other destructive microorganisms? Does immunity against invading and infectious microorganisms depend on a basic equilibrium of minerals?

When the clinical evidence of blocked lymph channels is present, noted in enlarged lymph nodes, it suggests the precipitation of iron due to the lack of the proper amount of potassium in the body. When this potassium is supplied lymph blockage disappears and lymph glands decrease in size.

I am constantly reminded of how much I owe the cows I have studied. When I made up my mind to go to school to them, so to speak, in order to find out the nature and practice of Vermont folk medicine, I decided not to try to tell the cows a thing, but to listen to them and let them tell me.

One herd of 45 registered Jersey dairy cows I studied illustrates the influence of potassium on invasion of the animal body by fungi and destructive microorganisms. Previously the amount paid annually for veterinary services for this herd was never less than $150.00. When potassium in its associated acid medium was started, with each cow receiving a total of four ounces of apple cider vinegar poured over its day's ration, it resulted in services of the veterinary being required only twice in the 14-month period of my studies. Apparently the added potassium maintained the body chemistry in a state which prevented invasion of the body by destructive microorganisms.

Wishing more proof, I decided to use the crows and foxes as censors at the first opportunity. This came when a cow in the herd began to lose weight and strength. She had an appetite and would eat, but apparently could not assimilate her food.

When the veterinary was called, he could not decide what was wrong, unless the cow was suffering a mineral deficiency. The cow grew weaker and finally died from starvation, as revealed by the autopsy requested by the veterinarian. No other disease condition was present, only the starvation.

I asked my friend, the owner of the cow, to have the carcass drawn to a hill on the farm where I knew there were fox holes. I had previously suggested that the animal might be helped by potassium, and it had been given to her in liberal amounts. Now I wished to observe the attitude of the crows and foxes to this potassium-saturated cow.

Ordinarily crows will descend on the carcass of a dead cow, to have a feast; to see them one would think it was convention time. But they kept strictly away from this carcass. The foxes kept away too. The outcome was that from February 11 to June 5 the carcass remained in full flesh. Then the maggots got to work and in a short time nothing remained but the bones.

When I came to study the relation of potassium to calcium I became interested in a herd of 54 cows in which one of the cows had enlarged knees. From difficulty she experienced on lying down and rising to a standing position, it was evident that her knees did not work well mechanically because they were inflamed. Along with the rest of the herd, she began receiving the two-ounce daily potassium treatment. At first there was no specific thought of influencing the size of her knees by use of the apple cider vinegar.

As time passed we noticed that she could lie down and get up with greater ease. At the end of a year both knees had returned to normal size. Naturally we questioned; could the potassium and acid in the apple cider vinegar have influenced the deposit of calcium favorably, and in both knee joints?

About this time a farmer came into my office to report his experience with a cow seven years old. The cow was stiff in the joints; it was painful for her to walk; she got up and down with great difficulty; a thickness had developed in the milk from one quarter of her udder—in fact, the milk was so thick that he could not get it out of the quarter with the milking machine.

In order to clear up the thick milk he poured two ounces of apple cider vinegar over her twice-daily ration. She liked the vinegar and lapped the manger after she had cleaned up her ration. The vinegar was stepped up to four ounces with each feeding. This not only cleared up the thick milk, it also cleared up the animal's arthritis, and she is now a normal cow. When she was started on the apple cider vinegar she was giving 11 pounds of milk a day; when she lost her arthritis, her production of milk went up to 32 pounds a day.

One day a farmer dropped in at the office to report on his arthritis. He said that before taking ten teaspoonfuls of apple cider vinegar to a glass of water with each meal he had had lameness in all the joints of his body. The first day after he began taking the mixture, his lameness was 20 per cent better and there was still more improvement the second day. By the fourth day he estimated a 50 per cent improvement, and at the end of a month a 75 per cent improvement. In addition to the lameness he had had pain in the joints, but that cleared up as the lameness lessened. Finally the pain cleared up altogether, including pain in the back of the head and neck.

I became very interested in the influence of apple cider vinegar on calcium metabolism in the animal and human body and began making calcium observations in order to better understand the results observed in arthritis.

Because of the large deposit of marble beneath the Vermont soil the drinking water in my part of Vermont, whether from spring or river, is very apt to be rich in calcium oxide. Indeed, so great is the amount of calcium that every two months calcium deposit has to be removed from the inside of a teakettle. People having an oil burner with a hot-water coil in the kitchen range have to purchase a new coil each year because the old one has become filled with deposited calcium. The large hot water tank in the building where my office is located deposits an inch of calcium on its inner wall every five years. In Vermont, people have learned by trial and error to remove deposited calcium on the teakettle by boiling up a solution in the kettle of one cup of apple cider vinegar to a quart of water. The deposited calcium goes into the solution in the boiling process and is disposed of when the teakettle is emptied. Sometimes more than one boiling is necessary.

I next studied methods used by plumbers in freeing the inside of the furnace water compartment from deposited calcium. When the water in the furnace would no longer boil quickly two quarts of apple cider vinegar were added to the water content of the furnace and allowed to remain for two days, by the end of which time the calcium had been dissolved and could be drawn off with the boiling water.

The above observations indicate that calcium enters into solution when the vehicle is acid in reaction. I then wanted to find out as to the condition under which calcium left a solution and was precipitated in the form of a deposit on the inside of a receptacle. When water was tested before boiling with Squibb's Nitrazine Paper, it was found to be neutral in reaction. After the water had been boiled it showed a very definite alkaline reaction. Apparently, then, calcium leaves a solution when it changes its reaction to alkaline, and enters a solution when its reaction is acid.

Here in Vermont each spring the precipitation of calcium in an alkaline medium is demonstrated in the making of maple sugar. Trees are tapped in the spring and the sap gathered. In the sugar house the sap is boiled until it has the consistency of maple syrup. Because of the marble deposit under the Vermont soil this sugar-maple sap is very rich in calcium, in the form of calcium malate. When the sap is boiled to make syrup this calcium malate is precipitated and forms what we call in Vermont "maple sugar sand." In order to remove this sand, the maple syrup is run through a felt

filter about a half inch thick. The point is that when the sap
is boiled, its alkalinity is sufficient to precipitate the calcium
malate.

One step in making a liniment commonly used in Vermont
folk medicine is to dissolve an eggshell in apple cider vinegar.
Place in a small glass jar the two halves of an eggshell. Now
add enough apple cider vinegar to cover them, and put the
top on the jar. Very soon, bubbles will begin to rise from
the eggshell to the top of the fluid. The outside of the shell
will soon be covered with many blisters of various sizes.
Within a day or two, the eggshell will have disappeared,
leaving behind a thin membrane. The calcium in the shell
has entered into solution in the acid medium represented
by the apple cider vinegar.

These five calcium observations have been outlined to
show that, outside of the body, calcium enters into solution
in an acid medium and is precipitated and deposited in an
alkaline medium. Have we any evidence that within the body
the fluid surrounding the body cells, represented by the
fluids of the blood and of the lymph between the body cell
walls, may increase its alkalinity, and in so doing present a
medium for the precipitation and depositing of calcium?

Medical literature tells us that the entire physiological
range of reaction of the extracellular fluid lies on the alkaline
side of neutrality. The blood represents one fourth of the
extracellular fluid. Its reaction is weakly alkaline. With an
alkalinity increased above its normal weakly alkaline reaction, calcium is precipitated and deposited in the tissues.

I became interested in knowing whether any change took
place when vegetables were boiled in water. With special
reference to my great interest in potassium, I sent to the
Package Library of the American Medical Association for a
package on "Potassium."

In the material received, I found a copy of the Proceed-
ings of the Staff Meeting, Mayo Clinic (12:424-432), July 7,
1937. I came across an article titled "Directions for the Plan-

ning and Preparation of Diets Low in Content of Potassium,"
by Sister Mary Victor, B.S., Fellow in Nutrition, The Mayo
Foundation. The article dealt primarily with the restriction
of the intake of potassium in Addison's disease. It presented
a list of foods high in potassium content which interested
me particularly because, with our Vermont topsoil low in
potassium content, we need to seek foods representing a good
source of potassium.

The list of potassium foods carried an interesting statement. "Values given for specially cooked vegetables were
obtained by analysis, after cooking. When cooked as described in a large volume of water, the reduction of potassium averages 70% in the case of carrots, kohlrabi, onions,
turnips, parsnips, potatoes, rutabagas, squash, pumpkin, and
spinach; 60% in the case of cauliflower, cabbage, peas,
asparagus, string beans, and brussels sprouts. The reduction
of potassium in corn, beets and tomatoes averages 50%."

We learn from experiments and the Mayo Clinic article
that a certain amount of calcium and potassium are lost when
the medium shifts its reaction from acid to alkaline. We have
evidence that potassium controls the use of calcium in the
body. If when a bone is broken it fails to unite, it can be
made to do so by the taking of one kelp tablet at each meal.
Kelp, as will be described more in detail later, is an excellent
source of potassium.

If you will drink a glass of cranberry or grape juice during
a meal you will find after the meal that your urine reaction
is now acid instead of alkaline. Your blood makes a complete circuit of your body every 23 seconds, and you have
flooded your blood with acid. By so flooding your blood
with a natural acid and the potassium it contains, any deposited calcium enters again into solution. This, repeated
day after day, keeps blood-vessel walls free from calcium
deposits.

In order to understand the relation existing between

potassium and sodium, we need to know that fluid inside the body cells represents 50 per cent of the body weight. The fluid in the blood represents 5 per cent of the body weight. The fluid which lies between the blood vessels and the cells represents 15 per cent of the body weight. We have then 50 per cent of the body fluid inside the cells of the body, and 20 per cent of body fluids outside the body cells. Both potassium and sodium have the ability to attract fluid. Within the body cells, potassium is responsible for drawing fluid into each cell. Outside the body cells, sodium is responsible for the amount of fluid present. Among our best sources of potassium are paprika, often sprinkled over salads; honey; fresh vegetables; fruit; and berries. Our best source of sodium is common table salt.

Potassium and sodium carry on a lifelong duel, fought over the supply of fluid. When sodium appears to be winning, a transfer of fluid from inside the body cells to outside the body cells takes place. When potassium appears to be winning, the transfer is in the other direction, from outside the body cells to within. An increased intake of sodium in the form of table salt will increase the loss of potassium from inside body cells, with the result that the body loses potassium. An individual cannot afford to lose potassium because it is the one mineral so necessary for proper performance by the nervous system.

Each individual who wishes to get the most out of life must learn to control his potassium-sodium balance. After all, since the body composition is partly mineral, an individual must become mineral-minded. By the way he feels during the day he can learn to tell what minerals his body needs to return his body to normal and, if he has lost it, to recover his body bounce.

CHAPTER **IX**

The Usefulness of Honey

MOST OF THE THINGS we do in life are the result of habit. Even our eating is largely habit. Native Vermonters have an ingrained respect for the nutritional wisdom of the bee, which goes into the fields and selects the materials for the making of a perfect food. With bees there are no new-fangled ways. By some infallible instinct the bee has some way of checking the quality of the flowers it visits to obtain nectar. It knows if and when flowers aren't up to its standards and moves along to others. In Vermont one sometimes hears the saying, "We've got to trust someone—why not let it be the bee?" The saying is more truth than poetry. Honey fills in any gaps that might occur in the daily food intake, and Vermonters take to eating it daily for that reason. People who know the food value of honey are more likely to eat it regularly than those whose knowledge of it is vague. A medical man who familiarizes himself with what honey can accomplish in the human body is very apt to prescribe it when rearranging the patient's daily food intake.

It is no mere theory but has been proved that bacteria cannot live in the presence of honey for the reason that honey is an excellent source of potassium. The potassium withdraws from the bacteria the moisture which is essential to their very existence.

At the Colorado Agriculture College in Fort Collins, Dr.

W.G. Sackett, a bacteriologist, determined to put honey to the test. He frankly did not believe that honey would destroy disease bacteria. So in his laboratory he placed various disease germs in a pure honey medium and waited. The results astounded him. Within a few hours' time, or at most in a few days, each of the disease microorganisms died. The typhoid-fever-producing germs died within forty-eight hours. Other similar germs called A and B typhosus, perished after only twenty-four hours. A microorganism found in bowel movements and water which resembled a typhoid bacillus died in five hours. Germs which caused chronic broncho-pneumonia were dead on the fourth day. It was the same with the particular bacteria associated with a number of disease conditions such as peritonitis, pleuritis, and sup-purative abscesses. Dysentery-producing germs were de-stroyed in ten hours. All these findings may be read in Bulletin No. 252, published by the experimental station where Dr. Sackett conducted his tests. Dr. Sackett was not alone in his experiments. These tests were duplicated and substantiated by Dr. A. P. Sturtevant, bacteriologist in the Bureau of Entomology, Washington, D.C.; by A. G. Lock-head, working in the Division of Bacteriology in Ottawa, Canada; and by numerous others.

There is recorded use of honey from cave-dwelling days. A bee's nest was found and some inquisitive soul tasted its contents of golden liquid. Liking the taste, he offered it to his family and when they were enthusiastic over it, he began to hunt systematically for places where bees stored honey and gathered it.

For ages honey made by the bees from flower nectars was the one food of pure sweetness available to man. In recent years there have been many substitutes for honey, in the form of manufactured sugars, tending to replace honey on our tables. Honey still remains the one sweet, however, offering life-giving qualities not found in any other.

In the light of the fact that the body has mineral requirements which must be met to establish and maintain good
health, let us examine the mineral content of honey. It is
important because most of us have only just begun to realize
that the diet of the average American is distinctly lacking in
needed minerals. We have become habituated to too many
foodstuffs that have been robbed of their natural mineral
content through processing and are therefore devitalized
when we get them. For this reason we need to know what
mineral shortages there are in the average daily food intake
and how minerals can be restored.

Iron, copper, manganese, silica, chlorine, calcium, potassium, sodium, phosphorus, aluminum, and magnesium are
all present in honey. They are all derived from the soil in
which plants grow, and are passed through by the plant to
the nectar which is the base substance used by bees to make
honey. Obviously, therefore, honey will vary in mineral
content according to the mineral resources in the soil where
its evolution starts.

In years gone by food authorities discounted the minerals
in honey, on the assumption that their quantity was too small
to make them important. Now it is known, however, that
numerous minerals are needed by the human body in very
small amounts to keep the body in mineral balance. Honey
contains them in about the right quantity to serve the needs
of the normal individual.

Professor H. A. Schuette, of the Department of Chemistry
of the University of Wisconsin, has this to say about the
mineral content of honey:

Of these newer essentials, copper, iron and manganese, there
seems to be a larger quantity in dark honeys than in light. From
a nutritional standpoint, iron is important because of its relation to the coloring matter of the blood, or hemoglobin. We
build hemoglobin out of our food, and it has a certain power,
carrying that all-important oxygen to our body tissues. Were it

not for its iron content, hemoglobin would not have this prop-
erty of holding oxygen.

Copper seems to unlock the therapeutic powers of iron, in
restoring the hemoglobin content of the blood in patients
afflicted with anaemia. In other words, copper promotes the action of iron.

We don't yet fully know the advantages of including manganese in the diet, but we do now know enough about the subject
to appreciate that it is a valuable adjunct to the diet. Some are
of the opinion that it functions more or less interchangeably
with copper, or as a supplement to it, aiding the formation of
hemoglobin in the blood. Others, however, hold that iron is
helped in this business of building hemoglobin by copper alone.
Yet they find also evidence in other connections to support their
opinions that manganese has a very specific function of its own
in nutrition.

What is the vitamin content of honey? Being a perfect
product of nature, it may be expected by definition to contain vitamins. The pollen of many flowers has a higher
vitamin C content than almost any fruit or vegetable. Honey
contains pollen. Obviously honeys with the largest amount of
pollen will have more vitamin C than others.

One of the most important facts established is somewhat
surprising, namely that honey is an excellent medium for
vitamins. This is not equally true of vegetables and fruits.
For example, spinach will lose 50 per cent of its vitamin C
content within twenty-four hours after being picked. Fruits
lose their vitamin content to a marked degree during storage.
Like most foods high in sugar, honey is low in thiamine but
fairly well supplied with riboflavin and nicotinic acid.
Nevertheless, honey contains all of the vitamins which
nutritionists consider necessary to health.

Whereas cane sugar and starches must undergo a process
of inversion in the gastrointestinal tract by the action of
enzymes to convert them into simple sugars, this has already
been done for honey by the bees, by means of the secretion

from their salivary glands, which converts the sugar in the nectar into the simple sugars levulose and dextrose, making it unnecessary for the human gastrointestinal tract to do this work. Thus does this predigestion of honey by the bee save the stomach additional labor. The fact that honey is a predigested sugar is not so important in a healthy human body which is capable of digesting sugar. It is very important when an individual has a weak digestion, or in an individual who lacks the two enzymes *invertase* and *amylase* to help the process of inversion.

Leaving aside as secondary the fact that honey is a welcome variation and delicious adjunct to the menu, it is a builder food, packed with the things the body needs to build and rebuild itself. It gives a quick energy release, which makes it appealing as a breakfast accompaniment to quickly give energy needed to start the day right. Let us count up the advantages of honey over other sugars:

1. It is nonirritating to the lining of the digestive tract.
2. It is easily and rapidly assimilated.
3. It quickly furnishes the demand for energy.
4. It enables athletes and others who expend energy heavily to recuperate rapidly from exertion.
5. It is, of all sugars, handled best by the kidneys.
6. It has a natural and gentle laxative effect.
7. It has sedative value, quieting the body.
8. It is easily obtainable.
9. It is inexpensive.

Yet for me the crowning glory of honey is its medicinal value. Being a medical man, I would naturally be interested in a substance which study and experimentation have convinced me is a help in living this life literally from the cradle to the grave.

Where else will I find for augmenting the daily food intake such a sedative as will calm down the nervous, high-strung, race-horse type of individual if taken at each meal, and doing only good, never harm, to the human body? Where will I find a sweet that will produce sleep at night?

Honey is soothing to the stomach. It will relieve an annoying cough. It has a laxative action which is effective, yet mild. It will relieve pain in arthritis.

I well remember the delight of a schoolteacher who reported what consistent use of honey had done for her arthritis. It had given her great pain for a long time and she had become quite philosophic about it. Then one year she was transferred to a new school district and went to board in a farm family. Honey was the standard sweetening agent used in the household. By the end of the teacher's first school year, the arthritis had disappeared. It could be attributed to the remedying of a potassium deficiency with the honey.

Honey will, by several effects, render old age less difficult to live. I am saddened when people tell me that they don't eat honey because it costs more than white sugar. I try to make them see that health is not to be had for the asking. Good health is earned. In the long run you must pay either the grocer or the drugstore. When you become sick, you find you must spend the money you saved on food to purchase drugs to bring back your health. By purchasing the right kind of food, such as honey represents, you can constructively cut some corners.

HONEY IN INFANT FEEDING

It is of course admitted that the normal mother's breast milk is the best possible food for her baby. But this natural food often becomes difficient in quality and quantity for the baby, especially as it grows older. It is then that modified cow's milk must be given in place of or to supplement mother's milk. Various sweetening agents have been used to bring cow's milk nearer to the requirements of the human baby. The sugars most commonly used for the purpose are *glucose* and *dextrimaltose*. Some recent work goes to show that honey, while more expensive than glucose, is still much cheaper than dextrimaltose, and superior to either for modifying cow's milk.

These days, many mothers seem unable to nurse their babies as Nature intended. This puts on the doctor the burden of compounding a diet suitable to the individual needs of the infant. Some infants, being very delicate, require infinitely careful handling. Some are allergic to certain foods while others are robust and seemingly can eat anything. The differences in toleration present problems which are difficult at times to solve.

The basis for all baby food but mother's milk is cow's milk, modified and sweetened. In this sweetening often lies the chief difficulty. The sweetener most often used is corn syrup, but many babies cannot tolerate this artificial sweetening agent. It becomes more evident every day that a natural sweet is much to be preferred to any manufactured sweet.

Honey is the outstanding natural sweet. Most babies can tolerate it and, in addition to being a sweet, it furnishes minerals supplementing those found in milk as well as a small amount of protein; it possesses an antiseptic, and a mild laxative, action; besides these advantages it has a fine flavor, which increases palatability. The chief factor is, of course, that it provides the infant with the composite of minerals needed for its growing body.

My own studies of honey in relation to baby food receive affirmative support in work done recently by Dr. M. H. Haycak and Dr. M. C. Tanquary of the University of Minnesota, and Dr. Schultz and Dr. Knott of the Department of Pediatrics of the University of Chicago. The following is taken from the work of Drs. Schultz and Knott:

In studying the comparative value of various carbohydrates in infant feeding, we employed honey along with other sugars.

Two groups of children were used to determine the effect of various sugars: four children from 7 to 13 years of age, and nine infants, ranging in age from 2 to 6 months. We fed the children diluted sugars, then took blood samples and determined the sugar content of the blood in 15 minutes after the meal, 30 minutes, 60 minutes, 90 minutes, and 120 minutes. When sugars are absorbed from the intestine, they enter the bloodstream and are carried to the liver to form glycogen. If carbohydrates are eaten above the limits of the liver to store them as glycogen, the excess is transformed in the tissues into fat, and stored as such.

Very interesting results are obtained with honey. During the first 15 minutes, honey was absorbed the most quickly of all the sugars tested, with the exception of glucose. Honey did not flood the bloodstream with an over-abundance of sugar. This response to honey is presumably due to the combination of the two easily absorbed sugars, dextrose, and levulose. Honey is taken into the body quickly because of its dextrose content, while the levulose, being somewhat more slowly absorbed, is able to maintain the blood sugar.

Honey has the advantage over sugars which contain higher levels of dextrose, since it does not cause the blood sugar to rise to higher levels than can be easily cared for by the body.

With its easy and widespread availability, palatability and digestibility, honey would seem to be a form of carbohydrate which should have a wider use in infant feeding.*

Because of these findings Dr. Schultz and Dr. Knott began to study the possibility of using honey as a sweetening agent in infant feeding. The remark at the beginning of their report on this work is worth mentioning:

Although honey has been known as a food from the earliest days of which we have historical records, its importance to man seems to have decreased as civilization advanced. In view of the fact that honey is a product ready for use without artificial treatment, and that it is composed of two sugars most acceptable to the body, it is strange that it has not enjoyed wider use, especially in the feeding of infants and children.

---

* "Use of Honey as Carbohydrate in Infant Feeding" by F. W. Schultz and E. M. Knott. *Journal of Pediatrics* (St. Louis, Mo., October 1938) 13:465-473.

In securing the many advantages of honey in infant feeding, one to two teaspoonfuls are used in eight ounces of feeding mixture. Should an infant become constipated, increase the amount of honey by one half teaspoonful. On the other hand, if looseness of the bowels develops, the amount should be decreased by one half teaspoonful.

Infants fed on honey rarely have colic; the rapid absorption of honey prevents fermentation from taking place.

I have assembled here some examples of conditions which I have found to be benefited by treatment with honey.

HONEY AND BED-WETTING

It may surprise some that Vermont folk medicine finds in honey a most efficient remedy for prevention of bed-wetting in children. When it continues after three years of age, bedwetting at night becomes a problem. Yet it is one of the most common conditions met with in children and is disturbing both to child and family.

For a very long time physicians, when asked what could be done to prevent bed-wetting at night, have replied that time would take care of it, the child would outgrow it. This indicated that no definite remedy was commonly known.

Symptoms of a habit of bed-wetting are clear-cut. In the majority of cases there is a common characteristic of frequent passing of urine during the day. As a rule these children are of the race-horse type, highly sensitive to stimuli such as excitement. The majority of children secure day control of the bladder before they are two years old, and by a few months later most of them are able to remain dry at night. Bed-wetting generally occurs every night, usually once or twice a night, and may begin after bladder control has been established. But it develops insidiously as a rule, as a continuation of the lack of control of the bladder at night which is present during infancy.

Some children wet the bed within an hour after going to sleep; with others it does not occur until the early morning hours. Some children awaken during the act or immediately following it; other children sleep through without interruption. On awakening in the morning there may be no recollection of bed-wetting but very often there are vivid dreams of convenience just before, or during, the act of bed-wetting; the sleeping child, instead of being awakened by the stimulation of the distended bladder, dreams that he is on the toilet or other place suitable for urination. These toilet dreams are so real that, upon being awakened, children will insist that they have gone to the bathroom.

Nearly always nervousness is present in children who wet the bed at night. In addition there may also be nail-biting, temper tantrums, thumb-sucking, and infantile speech.

Vermont folk medicine divides the treatment of bed-wetting into two parts: preventive treatment and active treatment. The preventive treatment is sometimes helpful. It consists in habit training for bladder control and should be started at about one year of age. The infant is placed on its toilet at regular intervals—such as on awakening, after each meal, and every three hours at first and at longer intervals as bladder capacity and bladder control improve—and encouraged to urinate. By the age of two years most children will tell those in charge of them when they desire to urinate.

In carrying out the active form of treatment, we seek a therapeutic agent which combines a marked ability to attract water and hold it, with a sedative effect upon the child's body. This treatment agent must be suitable for a long-range treatment program, and must be harmless to the child. It must be adaptable for continual daily use, or for use when needed only at certain times. Most important of all, it must be acceptable to the child. Vermont folk medicine finds these requirements are met in honey.

Honey, being hydroscopic, is able to absorb and condense

moisture from the atmosphere. The levulose in honey has the most moisture-attracting ability of any sugar. This moisture-absorbing ability of honey is readily observed in bread and baked pastries containing it, which will remain moist and palatable indefinitely. To make the most of this ability to absorb, condense, and retain moisture, honey should never be kept or stored in the refrigerator or the cellar; a dry and not too warm place and a tightly closed container are best suited to storing honey. One of the uses to which the moisture-attracting ability of honey can be put is to attract and hold the fluid in the child's body during the hours of sleep, so that bed-wetting does not take place.

However, supposing your child has the habit of bed-wetting at night. What would Vermont folk medicine have you do?

At bedtime give the child a teaspoonful of honey. It will act in two ways. First, it will act as a sedative to the nervous system. Second, as has been said, it will attract and hold fluid during the hours of sleeping. In attracting and holding the fluid it spares the kidneys.

As you continue using honey for this purpose you will learn when to use it. You will recognize conditions that are conducive to the difficulty. For example, attendance by the child at a children's party, with its accompanying excitement and liquid refreshments, will suggest the wisdom of a teaspoonful of honey at bedtime. Too, any increase in liquid intake, especially after five o'clock in the afternoon, will lead you to anticipate that an accident may occur during the night if nerves and kidneys are not protected.

When you have learned to control the situation with the honey at bedtime, begin to experiment by omitting it, to learn if it is not possible to establish normal night bladder control. You will soon learn the signs of the safe and unsafe nights. On what you recognize as the safe nights, you can try reducing the dose of honey at first, later omitting it. You will want to keep honey in reserve, to use when circumstances suggest an unsafe night. In any case it is a boon to nerves all around to know that such a simple measure as this use of honey is effective in ending an old difficulty.

USE OF HONEY IN PRODUCING SLEEP

A device much relied on by some people to induce sleep calls for lying with the eyes closed and visualizing a large blackboard. On the blackboard, you imagine your hand tracing with exquisite care, with a large paintbrush dipped in white paint, a big number 3. The number is traced very slowly, and when the first one is finished another is started. Most people are asleep by or before finishing the third. Another trick is to concentrate on relaxation of every joint in the body, finger joint by finger joint, to the wrist, up the arms, and so on, throughout the body. Many people find that this works.

Vermont folk medicine regards honey as the best remedy of all for producing sleep. If you should discover that you have difficulty in falling asleep at night, or that after you do go to sleep you wake up easily and find it difficult to get back to sleep again, you should make use of honey. If you take one tablespoonful of honey at the evening meal each day, you will soon discover that you are beginning actually to look forward to bedtime, and it may even become difficult to banish a feeling of drowsiness when for social reasons you may be up later than usual. You will observe the next morning that you must have fallen asleep very soon after your head touched the pillow.

It will not be quite as easy as this with everyone. If you find the one tablespoonful at the evening meal not quite enough to produce sound sleep, or something has happened during the latter part of the day to key you up, then make a mixture of three teaspoonfuls of apple cider vinegar to a cup of honey, and keep it on the night table in a wide-mouthed bottle or jar which will admit a teaspoon. Two teaspoonfuls of the mixture should be taken when you are preparing for bed. If you don't fall asleep within an hour, you will want to take two teaspoonfuls more. You can continue doing this at intervals of an hour for as long as necessary, but except for special circumstances you would probably not find more than two doses needful.

AN OLD-FASHIONED COUGH REMEDY

If you are troubled by a cough, make use of the following Vermont folk medicine cough remedy, which is many generations old here in Vermont and today works just as well as it has all these many years.

Boil one lemon slowly for 10 minutes. This softens the lemon so that more juice will be gotten out of it, and also softens the rind. Cut the lemon in two and extract the juice with a lemon squeezer. Put the juice into an ordinary drinking glass. Add two tablespoonfuls of glycerine; in terms of drugstore measuring, two tablespoonfuls equal one ounce. Stir the glycerine and lemon juice well, then fill up the drinking glass with honey.

Speaking of using lemons to compound a cough remedy, I recall the remark of a Vermont farmer. When he was explaining how well the suggested remedy had worked he laughed and said, "Fact is, we didn't have any lemons. I used apple cider vinegar. Just as good."

The dose of this cough syrup is regulated according to your needs. If you have a coughing spell during the day, take one teaspoonful. Stir with a spoon before taking. If you are apt to be awakened in the night by coughing, take one teaspoonful at bedtime and again during the night. If your cough is severe, take one teaspoonful on rising, one the middle of the forenoon, one after your midday meal, again in midafternoon, after supper and at bedtime. As the cough gets better, lessen the number of times you take it. I have observed several points which make it the best cough syrup

I know of. It does not upset the stomach, as many cough syrups do. It can be taken by children as well as adults. It will relieve a cough when all other cough syrups fail.

TO CONTROL MUSCLE CRAMPS, USE HONEY

At times we may be plagued by an annoying twitching of the eyelids or at the corner of the mouth. It can soon be made to disappear by the taking of two teaspoonfuls of honey at each meal. As a rule it will disappear within a week's time.

Cramps in the body muscles, which may appear from time to time, occur mostly in the legs and feet during the night. This muscle cramping can generally be controlled by taking two teaspoonfuls of honey at each meal. Generally it will disappear within a week and the honey should be continued indefinitely, for it is a way to prevent return of the difficulty.

HONEY FOR BURNS

In Vermont folk medicine, honey has long been used as a very successful treatment for skin burns. When applied it relieves the painful smarting and prevents formation of blisters. It produces rapid healing of the burned area.

EXPERIENCE WITH HONEY IN ATHLETIC NUTRITION

An article in the October, 1955, issue of the *American Bee Journal,* written by Lloyd Percival of Sports College in Canada and titled "Experience with Honey in Athletic Nutrition," presents very well "what native Vermonters who live close to the soil have learned about the use of honey." I would like to incorporate here a rather extensive section from Mr. Percival's conclusions because athletic sports are very important today in the schools and colleges, and athletic directors are constantly looking for ways of building strength, energy, and endurance in their squads.

Sports College has been actively interested in gauging the value of honey in athletic nutrition on an organized testing basis since 1951. Previously we had been interested in honey as an energy food, but had not done any organized or controlled testing to develop any specific knowledge. As is so often the custom, we had accepted it as a sound food, due to its wide acceptance. However, as our general research into such questions as ideal pre-activity meals, after-activity recovery aids, and methods of sustaining effort became an important part of our general operation, we became actively interested in finding out what were the foods and beverages that could be most helpful in these situations.

One of the questions we were most interested in was: What was the ideal energy food? We were interested in finding out what food, or combination of foods, would supply the greatest and quickest amount of energy, without causing digestive distress, or any other detrimental side reactions. In order to develop usable information, we organized a series of observation studies and tests.

We also started a campaign to collect information regarding the experience of others in the field of sports training and conditioning with the various energy foods and beverages. As a result of these tests and investigations, we now rate (a score rating of from 1 to 10) the popular energy foods and beverages as follows: Honey, 9; Glucose $7\frac{1}{2}$; Corn syrup, 7; Brown sugar 6; White sugar $4\frac{1}{2}$. In rating the popular energy foods we took into consideration the following factors: 1. Measureable reaction. 2. Digestibility. 3. Chemical reaction (acidity, etc.). 4. General tolerance of athlete to food concerned. 5. Caloric content per serving. 6. Taste appeal. 7. Versatility. 8. Economy. 9. Basic ingredients.

An analysis of our experience shows that: 1. Honey, as far as can be measured, supplies in an ideal way all the necessary energy requirements of the athlete for pre-activity fueling up; for the sustaining of effort during activity; for quick energy recovery after effort. 2. Honey, with its high caloric content, can build up energy with smaller servings. 3. It is extremely popular (by far the most popular) with athletes, due to its taste appeal. 4. More honey can be tolerated by the average athlete than any other of the energy foods and beverages tested. 5. Versatility makes it popular, since it can be used in many ways, and in combination with other foods and beverages. 6. It is a pure food, apparently free from bacteria and irritating substances.

As a result we recommend honey: 1. To be used in pre-activity meals. 2. For use after activity. 3. As a rest-period "jack-up" during activity. 4. In the daily diet, especially for breakfast, in order to supply daily energy needs. 5. As a general sweetener and spread. 6. In combination with such foods as fruit salad, yogurt, custards, rice pudding, etc. 7. As a baking and food preparation sweetener. 8. In making candy. 9. Generally, instead of other popular types of sweeteners.

Endurance: Athletes participating in endurance tests showed better performance levels when fed two tablespoonfuls of honey 30 minutes before the test began. Whenever honey feeding was withdrawn, there was a definite decrease in work levels accomplished. This was true in such tests as: Repeated running of 50-yard sprints, with 5-minute rest periods between such. Continuous running at a rate of 1 mile in 6 minutes. Swimming of repeated 100-yard sections, with 10 minutes rest between. *Note:* When a further feeding of honey was given at the halfway mark, work levels were increased.

Fatigue recovery: When given honey after a period of hard work, athletes recovered faster, and were able to continue working sooner. *Note:* Because of this reaction we have been advocating honey feeding for athletes who must study following hard practise or games. It has been our experience that honey feeding enables a student to study better, since his energy has been replenished.

Sustaining effort: Athletes fed honey during rest periods of hockey, basketball and football games, and between events in track and field, claimed they had greater energy and felt less fatigue during latter part of activity.

Hard Schedule: Athletes who had to play two games in two days reported they felt better in the second game when honey was used to replenish energy after the first game, and before the second.

Energy Lack: When athletes who had to practice or play after school or work (no food since lunch) took honey at lunch time, they reported disappearance of usual energy lack during activity.

Those reporting "energy lack" periods in mid-morning, reported great improvement when given honey as part of breakfast.

Weight Problems: Honey feeding (12 to 16 teaspoonfuls during day at meals and bedtime) prevented weight loss due to hard work, continued activity. When athletes were on a reducing diet, a teaspoonful of honey at the end of a meal gave a feeling of fullness, making diet less difficult, and helped them sustain feeling of vigor.

General conclusions: Sports College has no hesitation in saying that, because of the general experience with honey over a period of four years, honey is an ideal energy and fatigue recovery fuel. We recommend it for all athletically active people, and for all those who are interested in sustaining a high energy level throughout the day.*

THE HONEYCOMB TREATMENT

Honeycomb is excellent for treating certain disturbances of the breathing tract. The form in which it is used is the waxy comb substance from which all the honey has been abstracted. The value of chewing this honeycomb applies especially to the lining of the entire breathing tract. In addition to chewing the comb, eating honey each day is also part of the treatment. For this purpose comb honey is the first choice, but if for any reason comb honey is unavailable a tablespoonful of liquid honey as a dessert with each meal will produce desirable results.

As far as I have been able to learn, Vermont folk medicine uses honeycomb as a desensitizing agent, from the results obtained by its use it appears to be anti-allergic in its action. The compounding pharmacists are the honeybees, and Vermont folk medicine has unlimited faith in the wisdom of the honeybee.

* "Experience with Honey in Athletic Nutrition" by Lloyd Percival. *American Bee Journal* (Hamilton, Ill., October, 1955).

The observations of Vermont folk medicine relating to honeycomb would indicate that disorders of the breathing tract are deficiency conditions and, whatever the active principle is that is present in honeycomb, it is essential for the normal development and maintenance of the lining of the breathing tract.

I have not yet discovered the active principle in honey-comb. So far as I know, none of the drug companies that have studied honeycomb have yet been able to come up with the answer. I have, however, searched the available literature seeking a better understanding of both honeycomb and comb honey. From my reading I have learned that nectar gathered from the flowers by the honeybee is the chief source of carbohydrates which are converted into the easily digestible sugars dextrose and levulose. This converted nectar is called honey. In addition to dextrose and levulose there are found variable amounts of sucrose, dextrine, maltose, and other rare sugars, and also the minerals named earlier in this chapter. The acids found are formic, acetic, malic, citric, succinic, and amino. There are also carotin and x anthophyl pigments, albuminoids, and the enzymes invertase, diastase, catalase, and inulase. Honey also contains B complex com-ponents in micrograms per gram as follows: pantothenic acid 0.55, riboflavin 0.26, nicotinic acid 1.1, thiamine 0.044, pyridoxin 0.10, biotin 0.00066, folic acid 0.03.

Other food necessary to the honeybee is derived from pollen, which also is found in honeycomb. Chemical analyses of pollens have shown them to be rich in proteins and fats and to contain various carbohydrates such as sugar, starch, and cellulose. Beside the components specified as present in nectar, though the composition of pollen is by no means uniform, analyses of pollens gathered from various sources show wide variance in fats, starches, minerals and protein content.

Virgin scale wax, as secreted by the bees, is of uniform composition according to the U.S. Department of Agriculture

Bulletin E-495, February 1940. Its production has been found to follow the consumption of sugars only. Since this is true, it should be safe to assume that it contains at least some of the components of the nectar consumed.

The treatment results obtained with this combination of honeycomb and comb honey show a very high degree of efficiency. About 90 per cent of cases treated with the combination react very satisfactory within a few days' time, and often in much less time. Vermont folk medicine is authority for the finding that individuals who had comb honey in their diet until they reached their sixteenth year seldom have a cold, hay fever, or other nose disorders. It also teaches that the chewing of honeycomb creates an immunity to breathing-tract conditions that lasts for four years. It is reassuring to be able to add that, if comb honey has not been present in the diet up to the sixteenth year, results obtained indicate that it can be supplied at any time in later years and still produce the same normal functioning of the lining of the breathing tract.

During the period when honey made by the bees is being harvested you should seek out a beekeeper and get your year's supply of honeycomb, which the beekeeper refers to as *cappings,* for the reason that he must remove the cap of each honeycomb cell in order to drain out its contents of honey. If you should find that honeycomb cappings are too hard to chew comfortably, add some honey to them; it will soften them, making chewing easy.

Having spent considerable time checking this treatment, I should like to pass along some of the interesting things I learned.

Stuffy Nose

A boy eight years old was brought by his mother to my office for an examination and treatment of his nose. For five months he had had a continuous head cold which no treatment had favorably influenced. There was a profuse watery discharge and frequent nose-blowing was required.

This boy had had his tonsils and adenoids removed when he was three years old. Examination of his nose showed an appearance which would be present in hay fever—but it was too early for our Vermont hay-fever season. The mucous membrane in the nose was very pale and boggy in appearance. The boy breathed through his mouth because normal breathing was interfered with by a swelling in the nose tissues.

Following the general examination, and the special examination of his nose, I gave the boy a chew of honeycomb, to learn what might happen. I wrote out directions for treatment to be followed at home and prepared drops he was to take. Before I had finished this—after about five minutes—the boy suddenly said, "My nose is open! I can breathe through it!" I gave the medicine for home use to the mother and discussed the written directions. Then I examined the boy's nose again to see what the honeycomb had accomplished.

The nose tissues had subsided, as they would have if I had used a shrinking agent in the nose. Instead of being pale, the mucous membrane was now light pink in color. One week later, at the next office visit, the boy's nose was still open and he was breathing with his mouth closed.

In my office, at another time, I gave a woman with a large and very narrow nose one chew of cappings, to learn whether it would shrink down the nose tissues enough to enable her to breathe through her nose. The airway in each side of her nose was exceptionally narrow. At the end of five minutes she was able to breathe through her nose very much better, and this one chew of cappings kept her nose open for two weeks.

The chewing of honeycomb when a stuffy nose was present was tried with other patients, all with the same satisfactory results.

Nasal Sinusitis

The sinuses are an important part of the breathing apparatus, for they are connected to the nasal passageways and help to filter, humidify, and warm the air we breathe. Being hollow spaces in bone, they also affect the voice and lessen the weight of the skull.

There are eight sinuses, divided on both sides of the head. The maxillaries are located in the cheeks alongside the nasal cavaties. The ethmoids and sphenoids are behind the nose, near the base of the brain. The remaining two are the frontals; they are in the forehead above the eyes. These do not communicate directly with the nasal cavities, as do the other sinuses; they drain first to the ethmoids and from there to the nose. This makes them more difficult to treat because two, rather than one, sets of sinuses must be taken into consideration. The membranes lining these spaces are about one-25th of an inch thick, and are covered with a mat of fine microscopic *cilia*, or hairs. In this respect they resemble the inside of the nose, which has a similar lining. The hairs move to and fro like heat in the wind, and this movement propels mucus from the cavity. It is a most efficient self-cleansing arrangement.

When inflammation of one or more of the sinuses appears, it generally develops on an alkaline-urine-reaction background. When honeycomb is chewed the urine reaction is shifted from alkaline to acid, showing how quickly honeycomb brings about a change in body chemistry. So the individual with sinus trouble will want to remember which foods produce an alkaline urine reaction and avoid them until recovery from the sinus disturbance takes place.

The amount of honeycomb for one chew can be gauged by the ordinary chew of gum. Take one chew of honeycomb every hour for from four to six hours. Chew each amount for fifteen minutes and discard what remains in your mouth. If the sinus attack is acute, these four to six chews should bring about a disappearance of the symptoms in from one half day to a day's time. The nose will open up, the pain will disappear. Body energy will return and the sinuses will return to normal. It is well for one chew of honeycomb to be taken once a day for another week, to prevent any immediate recurrence of trouble. I would suggest further that if you care to take honeycomb in this way once a day from the time school and college open in the fall until the June closing and also take two teaspoonfuls of honey at each meal, in addition controlling your daily food intake, it will be very unlikely that you will have a repetition of sinus attack, an attack of influenza, or a head cold. My studies lead me to the conclusion that there is something in honeycomb which powerfully protects the breathing tract against sickness.

Hay fever

People who suffer from hay fever will assure you that there is no disease more dreadful known to man. Vermont folk medicine divides hay fever into three classes: mild, moderately severe, and severe. Its treatment is both preventive and symptomatic. If honeycomb cappings are chewed once each day for one month before the expected hay-fever date, the hay fever will either not appear or will be mild in character.

In mild hay fever the treatment taken once a day, on Monday, Wednesday, and Friday of each week, will keep the nose open and dry. If honeycomb is not available, take two teaspoonfuls of liquid honey at each meal.

Moderately severe hay fever should be treated by chewing honeycomb five times each day for the first two days, and three times a day thereafter for as long as needed. It is a good plan to eat comb honey each day if it is available; if not, the two teaspoonfuls of liquid honey, as sold at the grocery store, will prove effective.

In moderately severe hay fever the following has been observed:

1. Watery eyes would be dry in three minutes.

2. Stopped-up nose would begin to open in three minutes; in six minutes the nose would be clear for comfortable breathing with the mouth closed.

3. Running nose would be dry in five minutes.

4. Raw throat would be relieved in three to five minutes.

Where hay fever is severe, Vermont folk medicine advises the following:

1. Three months before the expected onset, take one table-spoonful of honey after each meal as a dessert. Comb honey is best but liquid honey will work; it is sometimes referred to as strained honey. Also take one tablespoonful of honey in one-half glass of water at bedtime.

2. Two weeks before the expected onset date, take a mixture of two teaspoonfuls of honey and two teaspoonfuls of apple cider vinegar to a half, or whole, glass of water, before breakfast and again at bedtime. This should be continued during your hay-fever season.

3. Continue taking one tablespoonful of honey after the mid-day meal, and supper as a dessert, at the same time keeping up the vinegar-and-honey mixture before breakfast and at bedtime.

4. If necessary chew honeycomb often enough during the day to keep the nose open and dry.

I have observed these results from this treatment. The vinegar-honey combination plus chewing honeycomb work better than hay-fever shots. Whereas the shots do not prevent the presence of mucus in the nose, there is no mucus when the Vermont folk medicine treatment is used.

Too, no matter how bad the hay fever is, with eyes and nose itching, when this treatment is followed there will be only a little sneezing and no watery discharge.

While I have not checked all these findings, I am told by those whose experience with Vermont folk medicine goes beyond my studies that the following results may be noted as early as the third day: 1. Sneezing stopped. 2. Dry eyes in three minutes. 3. Dry nose in five or six minutes. 4. Can pet the dog. 5. Can pet the cat. 6. Can feed the chickens. 7. Can milk the cow. 8. Can ride the horse. 9. Can sleep under wool blankets. 10. Can sleep on a feather pillow. 11. Can work in the flower garden. 12. Can cut ragweed. 13. Can smell the rose. Further results observed are that the chewing of honeycomb three or four times a week will eradicate hay fever in three years' time.

I have seen particularly interesting effects of this treatment in cases where work placed those who had suffered from hay fever in conditions regarded as extremely aggravating. For example, a high school boy worked on a farm. When the cows were fed late in the day it was his job to empty bags of grain into the herd feeding car. Every time he did this his nose would run water and block up and his eyes would pour forth water. He was given honeycomb to chew three times a day. By the end of one week he could do his job without any discomfort from nose and eyes.

Another high school boy who worked on a farm was experiencing very little trouble with his hay fever while he chewed honeycomb three times a day. 1 asked him to stop chewing it while he was in the midst of haying, so that we might test the responsibility of the honeycomb for freeing him of the hay fever. He did so. For seven days he remained free of it, even in the dust of haying. But on the eighth day his hay fever returned in all its old-time severity, and suddenly he was miserable. I started him up again on the honeycomb immediately. A week later I went out to the farm to see how he was getting along. He was on top of a hayload, storing the hay pitched up to him by the loader. I asked him how things were. "Fine," he grinned down at me. "No sneezing, clear nose all the time. No more time off from honeycomb for me!"

Lest the reader think these effective results are limited to Vermont, where the people have an ingrained experience with the remedies of folk medicine, I received information of an occurrence in Texas. An experiment in the treatment of hay fever was started in April, 1936, at William Beaumont General Hospital in El Paso. As the pollen season progressed from March to its height in August, so many cases of hay fever developed, and symptoms were so severe in El Paso and vicinity, that a public campaign was begun against the weeds responsible, and partially carried out in the city. Army personnel stationed here produced a heavy share of sufferers, and it was they who provided the stimulus for the experiment, together with one curious fact which came to light for the first time that year.

"Among the many home remedies for the treatment of hay fever which were brought up in discussion with the afflicted, one alone seemed of real value. Several individuals stated that in the past year or two they had received varying degrees of relief from symptoms by eating honey produced in their vicinity, and particularly from the chewing of the honeycomb wax." *

STICKY MATERIAL ON BUDS, AND RESINOUS MATERIAL ON BARK OF TREES

Many Vermonters, knowing of my studies in Vermont folk medicine, have called my attention to the sticky material present on plant buds and the bark of trees. Not long ago a man dropped in at my office, saying, "I couldn't bring you in a tree, but I found a branch split by wind in a storm and I thought you might like to have it. It shows spruce gum right well." The piece of branch is about a foot and a half in length, slightly concave. The inside curve has a "bubbled" appearance, with a profusion of gum "beads." He explained to me that spruce gum varies in color—brown, pink, or gray.

The sticky material is planned by Nature to protect the buds of plants and trees. Ants will seek out the sticky sub-

* "Time and Money Saved in the Treatment of Hay Fever" by Capt. George D. McGrew, M.C. U.S. Army. *The Military Surgeon,* May 1937. Col. 80, No. 5, pp. 371-72, 374.

stance on peony buds; wasps do the same. Honeybees are attracted to the sticky material on the bark of pine and spruce trees. When the Vermont farmer observes that his dairy cows eat plant buds for their sticky covering, and that goats do the same thing, he gets the idea that, when sickness comes to his own breathing tract, this sticky material will aid in restoring him to health, returning his breathing tract to normal.

So he gathers short, bud-bearing twigs from the pine tree, along with a few pine needles. He puts them in a dish, covers them with water, and lets them simmer slowly on the back of the stove for three days. During this time the water turns brown. This resulting brown liquid is run through a sieve and then thickened with honey. One teaspoonful of this mixture, taken several times a day, will end the sickness in the breathing tract.

Egg-shaped blisters are to be found on the bark of the fir tree. These blisters are punctured with a knife, and the liquid in them collected. A teaspoonful of this liquid taken three times a day will also clear up difficulty in the breathing tract.

CHAPTER **X**

The Usefulness of Kelp

THE ADVANTAGES OF CIVILIZATION are many, but it has its disadvantages also. The lack of mineral-bearing food is a major disadvantage. The composition of the human body being mineral, it is of utmost importance that it should be maintained by the needed minerals. Ocean kelp furnishes such a maintaining agent.

Sea water is water only in the sense that water is the dominant compound. It is a most complex liquid, containing about 3.5 per cent of dissolved inorganic compounds. Kelp, growing in the sea, converts these inorganic compounds into organic form.

Being the lowest portion of the surface of the earth, the ocean is the catch basin into which chemical substances of every kind have been dumped by the many moving forces in Nature. Loose and transportable materials are either moved directly and swiftly, or indirectly and by degrees, downward to the sea. Particles are carried bodily by wind, watercourse, and glacier. Other substances are dissolved in water and transported to the sea, where they are caught as it were in a trap and made permanently available. Thus has the ocean become a reservoir of accumulated wealth in chemical materials which makes the resources of the land appear insignificant by comparison.

This accumulation of useful materials is a direct challenge to chemists. It seems safe to predict that coming generations will learn the inexhaustibility of the ocean's hoarded wealth, and how to make priceless use of the complete assortment of chemicals it includes.

The surface area of the earth is 196,950,277 square miles. Of this area 70.73 per cent, or 139,295,000 square miles, are occupied by the ocean. The average depth of the ocean is estimated to be 2.38 miles, while the greatest depth yet found is 6.7 miles, in the Philippine Trench near Mindanao. More than four fifths of the ocean floor is covered by water more than a mile deep. Two thirds of it is covered by water 2 $\frac{1}{5}$ miles deep.

We do not know the composition of the first primitive seas. We do know, however, that throughout the ages many forces have been bringing material to the oceans from outer space, from the interior of the earth, and from the land. Meteors or cosmic dusts arriving on the earth have seven chances out of ten of falling in the ocean. Numerous rock meteors as well as those of iron and nickel are found strewn on the bottom of the sea. Volcanoes have contributed much to the ocean, either directly or by dust thrown high into the atmosphere, to be carried by wind over the ocean and brought down by rain. Submarine fissures and springs bring materials from the interior of the earth. Glaciers rasp out rocks, mud, and debris and, when they arrive at the shore, yield icebergs to drift to sea, where they melt and drop their cargoes of minerals.

Perhaps the greatest and most continuous addition to the ocean is carried by water. It is estimated that about .82 meter depth of water evaporates on the average over the whole ocean each year. This vapor, which is pure water with no minerals, rises in the air, is blown about the earth by wind, and is precipitated as rain. If we assume that 29.27 per cent of it falls on land, there is then 22 inches of rainfall over all the land of the earth. This water erodes and washes away the soil, which is carried as mud and silt down the brooks, creeks, and rivers back to the ocean. Part of it seeps into the ground to some depth, dissolving out soluble materials, issuing again in springs, geysers and artesian wells, and returning with its dissolved and suspended substances to the sea, where, again leaving its load of minerals in the ocean, it returns to the land for more. The most soluble substances go soonest and most completely. Whatever increases solubility also increases the impoverishment of the land and the enrichment of the sea. Among the most soluble compounds are the nitrates, the halogen compounds—the chlorides, iodides, bromides; also sodium, potassium, calcium, magnesium, and others. The less soluble substances, such as silica or sand, and the clays, or alumina, are left behind. It is these less soluble materials which are now the bulk of our soil.

Various agencies assist the process of escape of minerals to the sea. Every stroke of lightning oxidizes some atmospheric nitrogen to nitric acid, which is carried down by the rains to the soil, where it dissolves some minerals as nitrates. Some of this is used by plants, and some of it is dissolved and washed away to the sea. The carbon dioxide of the atmosphere dissolves in rain water and increases the solubility of limestone. Large quantities of this are transported down the rivers to the sea. While the above substances are carried in vast quantities to the sea, all minerals are soluble to some extent, though some of them more slowly; silica or sand, alumina, phosphates, and the like are carried in small amounts but add up over geologic time to huge quantities. The agencies of erosion—wind, frost, exposure to changes of temperature and sunlight—all tend to aid the escape of substance from the land to the sea. Mountains and hills slowly crumble, valleys are chiseled out, rocks disintegrate and decompose and are dissolved and washed away.

Man himself has been a party to the robbery of the land. The primitive forest, with its leaves, roots, and vines, held the soil in place and served to restrain the flow of water to some extent and to prevent direct erosion of the soil. Now that man has cleared away the forest and laid bare the ground, solid substance is carried away much more rapidly than ever before. In more primitive times man returned sewage, wastes, and dejecta to the soil. Now he has become sanitary and discharges what came from the soil into the rivers, and eventually into the ocean.

Man is also digging iron, tin, copper, zinc, and other minerals from the ground, making them into automobiles, tin cans, buildings, and so on. Eventually these are worn out, discarded, piled up in junk heaps, there to rust, corrode, burn, dissolve, and wash away finally to the sea. Vast quantities of materials are destroyed by combustion as fuel, or for disposal of wastes. All of the coal, most of the petroleum, and much of the products of forests are eventually consumed by fire. Their smoke and dust go into the air, their ashes are leached out by rain, the portable materials going to the sea.

The various materials, upon entering the ocean from the rivers, begin at once to take part in a vast milling of chemical changes, reacting, dissolving, precipitating, redissolving, being taken up by living plants and animals, going through the life cycle and being set free again. Almost every kind of reaction has a chance to occur because the ocean is forever stirred by wind, and currents horizontal and vertical, exposed to change of temperature, frozen and thawed, exposed to light of varying intensities and colors. As it now exists the composition of the ocean is the result of millions of years of these reactions. Everything that exists anywhere in the earth or above it finds its way at last into the sea. Every element necessary for life is present everywhere in the sea. Sea water and healthy human blood have an almost identical chemical constituency.

In the sea there is and can be no deficiency. Every element necessary for life is present everywhere, and the living animals and plants of the ocean select what they require. Seafoods are capable of supplying all the elements necessary in our foods, whether we know what they are or not. In seafoods the necessary elements not only have been selected and assimilated on the basis of the natural requirements of living tissues, but they are stored and available in the form of a natural food in something approaching the proper proportions of the diet of man.

Chemists have known for centuries that in the vast ocean there are dissolved almost all the important chemical elements. It is estimated that each cubic mile contains about 200,000,000 tons of chemical compounds including elements like gold, silver, magnesium, aluminum, radium, barium, bromine, iodine, sulfur, and many others. With knowledge that the ocean serves as a mixing bowl for the mineral elements washed from the land, it is readily understood why marine plants and animals face no deficiencies. In time they take these mineral elements and assimilate them into organic combinations which are, in turn, needed by land inhabitants to prevent and cure deficiency diseases. Life reaches its richest abundance and its most varied forms in the sea. From small creatures invisible to the naked eye—teeming millions of them in a cubic inch of water—to the great whales, runs the animal life of the sea. Its tropical and semi-tropical waters are layer upon layer of life communities, starting at the very bottom of the sea and extending to the surface.

Equally rich in abundance of form and size with the sea's animal life is its plant life. It too starts with tiny forms visible only with the microscope and continues up to the great tree of the sea, the giant kelp.

Feeding in their marine pasture, sea animals are supplied with food so abundant, so rich in vital elements, that their rate of increase is many times greater than that of land-dwelling creatures. Why does life flourish so much more abundantly in the sea than on the land? Why are people whose diet includes much seafood practically free from certain disturbances to which others are subject?

The answer lies in the completeness of the sea's supply of mineral matter needed for health. Sea plants grow in a mineral-rich medium. They take from this source and store up these important minerals. When seafood, either plant or animal, is eaten, these minerals are reabsorbed and perform their marvelous chemical functions of regulation and correction. The numerous elements coming from the sea, one of the most important of which is iodine, furnish the final essential link in the balanced diet.

The most essential mineral elements of the body composition, in the order of their apparent importance, are iodine, copper, calcium, phosphorus, manganese, sodium, potassium, magnesium, chlorine, and sulfur. All but the first of these, iodine, which is a native of the sea, have their source in the soil. We would naturally suppose that when we eat products of the soil we should secure an ample supply of them. That is no doubt what Nature intended. But Nature did not foresee that man would remove the trees and other growth, allowing the rains to erode the soil, leaching out the essential minerals and, by means of our creeks and rivers, carrying them down to the sea. The result has been mineral-starved soils, in turn producing mineral-starved foods. The obvious result is that humans, who depend upon these mineral-starved foods for our supply of minerals, are literally starving in the midst of plenty.

It is easy to know when one is hungry for sweets, starches, or fats. The body sends out distress signals almost immediately and, if we are in normal health, our appetite tells us what is needed.

Once we learn to know them, the signs of mineral hunger are quite as definite and the results, if our body's SOS is long ignored, are far more serious.

There have developed within the last few generations, especially here in the United States, where food is most abundant and the average person eats most generously, a whole series of "deficiency diseases." It is recognized that each of these diseases is due to a lack of vital elements in the diet, and the essentials most often lacking are the essential minerals. The thyroid requires iodine. The parathyroid requires cobalt and nickel. The adrenal glands require magnesium. The pancreas requires cobalt and nickel. The anterior pituitary gland needs manganese. The posterior pituitary needs chlorine. The gonads require iron.

An entirely new respect is being acquired for iron, copper, manganese, zinc, and aluminum, for it has been discovered that these minerals have a most profound influence as catalysts, or electrifiers, or self-starters, in our body processes in general and upon the formation of good and plentiful blood in particular.

Iron enters directly into the construction of the hemoglobin of red corpuscles, which are the oxygen carriers of our blood. Anemia is a deficiency disease which may develop if there is an insufficient supply of iron in the blood. Unfortunately the human body cannot store up much iron, so it is necessary to replenish the supply regularly.

Though our diets are mineral-deficient because the soil is mineral-starved, fortunately we know where these mineral riches have gone. Every year, every day, as our soils become more impoverished, the seas become richer in these minerals. So we are learning to do a quite natural and undoubtedly a very wise thing—we are going back to the sea for the minerals of which our lands have been despoiled. We are appreciably developing a new interest in seafoods, but—as sparingly as we consume sea foods as yet—it is still difficult to catch up by the use of seafoods alone with our clear lack of minerals.

However, we find in the ocean a plant whose botanical name is *Macrocystis pyrifera* and which is commonly called *kelp*. It is often referred to as a sea vegetable and serves well as a food supplement.

Kelp grows in great abundance off the California coast. It

flourishes best at a depth of from six to ten fathoms and is found only where the ocean bottom is rocky. It has no roots but is anchored to the rocks by tough ropelike cables, called *hold-fasts,* and derives its nourishment entirely from the water. It is one of the largest plants in existence, often reaching a length of seven hundred feet, growing as much as fifty feet in a single year. Each plant consists of a trunk or stem, lined on either side with large single lanceolate leaves. The leaves occur in files of six or eight or more, the files alternating, each leaf supported by a buoy or floater at its point of contact with the trunk of the plant. Each leaf is finely but irregularly corrugated, is bordered with a single row of short, soft spines, and is olive brown in color.

Biochemistry teaches us that plants are the only organisms that can manufacture food, and that the essential food elements man receives from the flesh of animals come originally from plants. As every raw material essential for plant life is right at hand, the seaweeds such as kelp are naturally rich in the food elements required by man and other forms of animal life. The minerals it absorbs from the water in such abundance are present in an organic colloidal state, readily usable, and directly transferrable to the human body.

Heretofore most peoples have availed themselves of the vast food supply of the sea as created only indirectly, through the consumption of fish and certain crustaceans. Some maritime nations, however, like the Japanese, the Irish, and formerly our coastal Indian tribes, have been large consumers of edible seaweeds. It should be noted that, because of this diet, certain deficiency diseases have been very rare or entirely absent among these peoples. For example, the natives in Japan eat about the equivalent of ten grains of dried kelp each day; in the Japanese boats coming to California there are always six or seven different varieties of kelp stored in the supply room to be eaten later.

I asked the late Professor Cavanaugh of Cornell University where one might obtain kelp that was carefully prepared so that it might safely be given to patients. He said that the kelp he used in experimenting on farm animals, poultry, and in tablet and granular form for human consumption was obtained from Philip R. Park, Inc., of San Pedro, California.

Happening to be in California to attend a medical meeting, I visited the plant of this company. I wanted to familiarize myself with the manner in which kelp was harvested from the ocean and the method of its preparation for the consumption of humans and farm animals.

A couple of harvesters gather the kelp from the sea. They operate off the shores of San Clemente Island and in the kelp beds between Redondo and the San Pedro Breakwater.

The kelp harvester is an interesting contraption. It operates at the end of a barge onto which carriers load the kelp as it is cut. The harvester works something like a mowing machine, but in addition to the horizontal blade it has a vertical blade on either side. The cutting apparatus is lowered into the water to a depth of three feet and shears off the tops of the kelp plants. The government does not permit it to be cut more than that much.

The larger of the harvesters mows a swath 18 feet wide and gathers a load of two hundred tons in six hours. It is operated by a gasoline engine at the farther end of the barge.

The kelp is unloaded at the factory by means of a couple of huge iron forks, which are operated by a crane and which clasp the kelp like the fingers of two hands. They pick up as much as nine hundred pounds of kelp at one time and dump it into a hopper, where it is cut up in less than a minute. From the cutter it passes on a conveyor to a macerator, in which it is reduced to a pulp, and then run into a huge storage tank. A pumping system conveys it from this tank to the drier.

At this stage the kelp flows quite readily. Its water content, together with the ooze that attaches to the plant and makes it extremely slippery, mixed with the fine pieces of kelp produces a maze of semiliquid pulp of a consistency like that of heavy gruel. In the drier the process is so controlled that the constituent elements of the kelp are preserved.

The drier, of which this firm has three, is a revolving steel tube 60 feet long and six feet in diameter. At the end of the tube where the macerated kelp enters is a gas furnace, which provides the heat. This end is several feet higher than the other end. At the lower end is a large fan. The incline of the drier, its revolutions, and the current of air produced by the fan cause the kelp to move slowly through the tube while the dehydrating process is going on. In its course it passes through heat ranging from 1400 degrees Fahrenheit at the entrance to 300 degrees at the point of exit.

When it emerges from the drier the kelp is in small pieces, somewhat like fine popcorn. It is then run through a grinder and comes out in the form of a coarse powder. In this condition it is ready to take its place in the preparations manufactured by the company.

The company has a large, well-equipped laboratory containing a large number of rabbits, hens, and white rats to which its kelp preparations are fed. A minutely accurate tabulation is made of the results in every important aspect. The company prepares a 5-grain tablet form of kelp for human consumption and the seaweed is also prepared in granular form.

A number of years ago the late Dr. Weston A. Price of Cleveland, Ohio, internationally known for his work relating to the cause of dental decay, came to Barre to discuss with me my years of study of native Vermonters living close to the soil, and of Vermont folk medicine. He had just returned from a trip to Peru, where he studied and photographed the condition of the teeth of individuals living at high altitudes in the Andes Mountains. He had been all over the world studying the teeth of primitive peoples, in an effort to learn causes of dental decay, and wished to add to his studies dental conditions of people living in high altitudes.

He himself was unable to go higher than 12,000 feet, but

he learned about individuals living at 16,000 feet. He arranged for some of them to be brought down to 12,000 feet so he might study them and photograph their teeth.

While he was working he chanced to notice that each individual carried a little bag, of which all seemed to be particularly careful. Out of curiosity he looked into the bags and discovered that they contained kelp. When he asked where they had got kelp so far from the ocean, they said calmly that they got it from the ocean. This surprised him since it took a month to make the trip to and from the coast. What did they use the kelp for? To guard the heart, they explained to him.

Soon after Dr. Price visited me a patient who had had several heart attacks came to my office to have his ears inflated. He came on a Friday and I asked him to return on the following Monday. He said he did not know whether he could make a second visit because, in climbing the one flight of stairs to my office, he had been obliged to stop and rest three times because of pain in his heart. He said that he was obliged to remain quiet throughout each morning so that it would be possible for him to be moderately active in the afternoon and evening.

I gave him some 5-grain kelp tablets with instructions to take one tablet either before, during, or after each meal, whichever he found most convenient.

The following Monday he walked into my office and, holding out his wrist, asked me to take his pulse. It was 72 for the minute count. I then asked why he had wanted me to take it. He said that since taking the first kelp tablet he had been completely free from heart pain. He had walked up the stairs on this second office visit without having to stop and rest. I had him continue taking one 5-grain kelp tablet at each meal, with the result that he became much more active than he had been.

A minister and his wife who lived in California were visiting at our home. During the course of conversation an expression indicative of severe pain came across his face, and he clutched his heart region with his right hand. When we were alone I asked him if he had suffered pain in the heart and he said he had. Occasionally he would have this momentary heart pain and he was quite concerned about it.

I told him about Dr. Price's experience with the Peruvian natives living at 16,000 feet and gave him some kelp tablets with instructions to take one tablet at each meal. I learned later that this ended the attacks.

At Cornell, Professor Cavanaugh showed me his experimental work with kelp on white Leghorn hens, which demonstrated how much their health could be improved by a food supplement in the form of sea kelp and how much better the eggs were. He demonstrated how hard the shells of the eggs were and how the egg yolk could be tossed from one hand to the other without breaking. He was particularly interested in preventing soft-shell eggs.

Professor Cavanaugh also discussed cases of un-united bone fractures which medical friends had talked over with him, asking what was wrong with the body chemistry that prevented formation of new bone and what was needed by the body in order to bring about bony union. In each case, he suggested, patients should be given kelp tablets, which he recommended strongly because it was such a good source of the minerals in organic from which the body needed. Later reports to him said that bony union took place promptly after the kelp treatment was begun. Later Professor Cavanaugh made a study of the influence of kelp on the healing time of fractures when kelp was taken each day. Determinations were made of the blood calcium, phosphorus, iron, and iodine on patients with fractures at different intervals during convalescence. This study disclosed that the healing time of fractures could be reduced 20 per cent by having the patient take kelp each day and that kelp raised the blood calcium.

The composition of the human body and the composition

of seven gallons of sea water are the same. In view of this fact it would seem practical to turn to the sea in order to supply the mineral needs of the body. To a certain extent we are already doing this, by eating fish and other seafood grown in the ocean. We shall materially step up the process if we take one 5-grain kelp tablet each day. This is a simple, effective means of avoiding the mineral-deficiency conditions which appear in the human body when we eat only land-grown foods, which all too prevalently are grown in mineral-starved soil.

Many native Vermonters who have left the state to live at other points along the New England coast have reported the regular gathering of kelp washed up on shore after a storm. They dry the kelp and crush it with a rolling pin. They make a dessert of it by adding a teaspoonful of the crushed kelp to each cup of water. The mixture is allowed to simmer on the stove until it has the consistency of strained honey. After being taken off the stove and allowed to cool, whipped cream is added and it is served for dessert.

Moss is also used, pulled from seacoast rocks when the tide is out. This is dried and eaten without cooking. For many years I have seen a seaweed called dulce sold in the grocery stores of Barre. It is very much favored and I deduce that kelp and these similar marine substances must present something which the body very greatly desires, or they would not be in such regular use.

CHAPTER XI

The Importance of Iodine

FOLK MEDICINE IN VERMONT is interested in three R's— Resistance, Repair, and Recovery. First the individual asks himself whether his resistance to disease is as it should be. Next, is he able to repair tissue injury due to accident should it occur? Finally, if sickness should come, is his body able to bring about recovery?

Somehow during the passing years he has learned that iodine is related to the ability to resist disease.

Iodine is necessary for the thyroid gland's proper performance of its work. The human thyroid gland is located in the front of the lower part of the neck. All the blood in the body passes through the thyroid gland every 17 minutes. Because the cells making up this gland have an affinity for iodine, during this 17-minute passage the gland's secretion of iodine kills weak germs that may have gained entry into the blood through an injury to the skin, the lining of nose or throat, or through absorption of food from the digestive tract. Strong, virulent germs are rendered weaker during their passage through the thyroid gland. With each 17 minutes that rolls around they are made still weaker until finally they are killed *if* the gland has its normal supply of iodine. If it does not, it cannot kill harmful germs circulating in the blood as Nature intended it should.

It is well established that the iodine content of the thyroid gland is dependent upon the iodine available in the food and water intake of the individual. If the iodine intake is low the gland is deprived of an element it needs to do its work.

We learn in Vermont folk medicine, however, that this gland performs other functions besides killing harmful germs in the blood. The first is the rebuilding of energy with which to do the day's work. There is a definite relationship between the amount of energy you have and your iodine intake. The first question in the presence of a condition of depleted energy is, Is the soil of the state in which one lives iodine-poor? Second, is the deficiency being made up by supplementary means? All soils containing granite are iodine-poor and Vermont is one of them. This fact is very important to people living in Vermont and well may be important to those living elsewhere. When energy and endurance run low in relation to doing the day's work, then the taking of iodine needs to be considered.

A second function of iodine is to calm the body and relieve nervous tension. When nervous tension runs high there is irritability and difficulty in sleeping well at night, and the body is continually on a combat basis, organized for fight and flight. All these points stress a body need for iodine to lessen nervous tension, relax the body and enable it to organize for peace and quiet, by the building and storing of body reserves against time of need. I have learned through Vermont folk medicine that it is possible to repeatedly change an irritable, impatient, and restless child under ten years of age into a calm, patient individual within two hours' time by giving one drop of Lugol's solution of iodine by mouth in a vegetable or fruit juice or in a glass of water made acid in reaction by adding a teaspoonful of apple cider vinegar. I have repeatedly prescribed this in order to make it possible for a mother of a racehorse-type little boy or girl to be able to live comfortably with the child. I have never seen it fail to calm down a nervous child.

A third function of iodine in the human body relates to

clear thinking. The mind simply works better when the body is supplied the iodine it needs.

Then there is the matter of the storing of unwanted fat. Iodine is one of the best oxidizing catalysts we have. A catalyst is the match which touches off in the body the fire that burns up the food we take in each day. If this food is not properly burned off, it may be stored as unwanted fat.

Now while the thyroid gland helpfully stores iodine from the blood passing through it every 17 minutes, the gland may also be made to lose that stored iodine if, for example, we take in drinking water to which chlorine is added, or use too much sodium chloride, whose common name is table salt.

There is a well-known law of halogen displacement. The halogen group is made up as follows:

Halogen	Relative Atomic Weight
Fluorine	19.
Chlorine	35.5
Bromine	80.
Iodine	127.

The clinical activity of any one of these four halogens is in inverse proportion to its atomic weight. This means that any one of the four can displace the element with a higher atomic weight, but cannot displace an element with a lower atomic weight. For example, fluorine can displace chlorine, bromine and iodine because fluorine has a lower atomic weight than the other three. Similarly, chlorine can displace bromine and iodine because they both have a higher atomic weight. Likewise, bromine can displace iodine from the body because iodine has a higher atomic weight. But a reverse order is not possible. A knowledge of this well-known chemical law brings us to a consideration of the addition of chlorine to our drinking water as a purifying agent. We secure a drinking water that is harmful to the body not because of its harmful germ content but because the chlorine content now causes the body to lose the much-needed iodine.

Because we may live in an iodine-poor area; because drinking water may be treated with chlorine; because we may be sick too often, lack energy and endurance, develop nervous tension, lack the ability of clear thinking, and accumulate unwanted fat, how shall we go about bringing up the iodine content of the body to the point needed?

There are three ways:

1. Eating foods which analysis has shown are particularly rich in iodine. Among these are: all food out of the ocean, radishes, asparagus, carrots, tomatoes, spinach, rhubarb, potatoes, peas, strawberries, mushrooms, lettuce, bananas, cabbage, egg yolk, and onions.

2. Painting a small area of the body with tincture of iodine.

3. Taking preparations known to be rich in iodine. One of these is cod-liver oil. Another is Lugol's solution of iodine, which can be purchased at the drugstore. Still another is the kelp tablets hirtherto discussed.

The Lugol's solution is an inexpensive preparation to take. In 1880 a French physician named Lugol originated a solution which contains 5 per cent of elemental iodine in a 10 per cent solution of potassium iodide. It has been used steadily ever since it was originated. Every pharmacist knows how to make Lugol's solution. If he doesn't have the time to make it, he orders it from his wholesale drug supplier. Every drugstore carries it in stock. Here in Barre it sells for less than a dollar an ounce.

When used to maintain the iodine content of the body the dose is small and is taken only on certain days of the week. When the mineral content of the body is analyzed, only a trace of iodine is found. Ten drops of iodine represent more iodine than is found in the entire body. For this reason, the dose of Lugol's solution of iodine is one or two drops, depending on your body weight. If you weigh 150 pounds or less, for example, your dose to maintain the normal iodine content of the body is one drop, taken at one meal on Tuesday and Friday of each week. If you weigh more than 150 pounds, the dose should be two drops instead of one. It is useful to remember that the human body works on the minimum of anything it needs. If there should be a rise in sickness in the area where you live, it would be well to take the Lugol's solution three times a week instead of two, on Monday, Wednesday, and Friday, for the purpose of storing up reserve.

How is the drop of the solution to be taken, on the directed days? In general, medical men prescribe iodine to be taken on an empty stomach, preferably 20 minutes before food is taken.

During the passing years Vermont folk medicine has worked out a different plan and it is one I like to follow. It has been referred to in another connection elsewhere in this book. To repeat, adding one teaspoonful of apple cider vinegar to a glass of water to make the water acid in reaction, holding the medicine dropper horizontal in order to get a maximum drop, one drop of the Lugol's solution is added to the mixture. The contents are stirred with a spoon and sipped through the course of the meal, as one would drink a cup of coffee or tea.

In relation to supplemental use of iodine, my studies of certain dairy herds has revealed interesting evidences of the relationship between host and microorganisms, viruses, insects, and other parasites.

With one herd the veterinary bill had generally run $150.00 and sometimes more a year. At my suggestion, three drops of Lugol's solution of iodine was added to the daily four ounces of apple cider vinegar. Thereafter it was only necessary to call the veterinary once in a period of eight months, to see a sick cow. In contrast to this, another herd, to which Lugol's solution was not given, had plenty of sickness. In an 8-month period it was necessary to spend $50.00 for penicillin in order to save seriously sick cows.

I have observed that lice will leave the hide of a cow that receives apple cider vinegar and iodine; also that flies will not bite the cows when they are on pasture, though flies will and do bite young cattle not receiving the apple cider vinegar and iodine.

In a herd troubled with abortions—evidence of the work of the *Brucella abortus* microorganism which grows on a alkaline medium and causes contagious abortion in catt called Bang's disease, or *brucellosis*—abortions promptl stopped when each feeding ration received a supplementa three drops of Lugol's solution of iodine to each two ounces of the apple cider vinegar.

While studying selected herds, I became interested in the problem of cattle grubs. These are the larvae, or maggots, of the heel fly. The adult fly does not bite or sting, but it produces great fear and is a serious annoyance to the cattle. Eggs are deposited in a row attached to a single hair of a cow's heel during the first sunny days of spring. The eggs incubate and hatch in three or four days and the newly hatched maggots penetrate the hide of the cow, causing itching and a flow of serum that mats the hair. The young grubs then work their way upward between the muscles and may be found in a few months in the body cavities. They continue to burrow along the surface of the paunch, intestines, and other internal organs. At certain times many of them are found in the wall of the esophagus, leading from the mouth to the stomach. During the fall and winter the grubs will finally come to the top of the back and lie just under the hide. Each grub cuts a hole through the hide to the surface to get the air which it now needs, and to permit it to escape when ripe. The period spent beneath the hide usually runs from 30 to 90 days. These grubs emerge from the hide during February and March, dropping to the ground to hatch into heel flies. In 18 to 80 days after escaping from the back of the cow, the adult fly hatches and is ready to mate within a half hour.

My object was to rout these cattle grubs by means of the apple cider vinegar and iodine combination; this would demonstrate, to me at least, what the combination would do in the way of making the body as a host unsuitable soil for the development and continuing existence of microorganisms, viruses, insects, and other parasites.

During one year's time only ten grubs were discovered on the backs of a herd of 45 registered Jersey cows. Usually these grubs are a little larger round than a pencil, but these ten grubs had such hard going in the cows' bodies against the vinegar and iodine that they were no larger around than toothpicks. I observed further with reference to a ration supplement high in iodine value that when it was used, the bacterial count of the milk went down; when iodine was discontinued, the count went up but could be driven down again immediately with resumption of the iodine.

From Dr. William Weston of South Carolina and his experience with race horses wintered there, I gained interesting and valuable insight into the value of iodine in the body, and its relation to endurance.

About 100 race horses are wintered where he lives. Two years previous to a visit I paid him, the man in charge of the horses came to him saying that a horse was under his care which had everything it takes to win the Kentucky Derby. If they could just learn precisely how to feed this horse to maintain its speed capability, he believed the horse would have an outstanding racing season. Would Dr. Weston help him by planning the feeding of the horse?

Dr. Weston was greatly interested and consented to do so. As a first step he asked for samples of any and all foods given the horse. The samples were analyzed at the South Carolina Food Research Laboratory. As a result of the analysis, Dr. Weston advised increasing the iodine content of the ration, by incorporating into it foods specifically rich in iodine.

This was done. In the ensuing season the horse won every race in which it was entered.

As a result of the experience, two wealthy race-horse owners invited Dr. Weston to come to their horse farms to discuss the feeding of their stock. Again iodine-rich foods were added to the usual rations, with the same result; every horse fed on iodine-rich diet won every race in which it was entered. This seems to be a complete demonstration of the relation of iodine to energy and endurance.

Subsequently, Dr. Weston sent me a copy of a letter addressed to him as chairman of the South Carolina Food Research Commission. It well illustrates the need of observing the obligation to Nature which must be observed by a daily intake of iodine. The letter ran as follows:

Dear Dr. Weston:

Now that we have reached the halfway mark of this racing season, I should like to tell you some of our observations of the results of wintering our horses in South Carolina, and feeding them your home grown feeds.

After six years of experiment with several hundred horses, we are more convinced than ever that your foods, abundant in iodine and balanced in mineral content, are the saving factor in many of our horses. Allow me to give you an example. This summer an epidemic of influenza and coughing broke out among two year olds at the New York tracks. It spread like wildfire through the stables, and all the old cures and preventives were useless against it.

We have checked carefully and find that none of the horses that were wintered in South Carolina, were affected. Naturally we spoke of this often, and by so doing attracted the attention of many people to South Carolina, and the merits of your theories and findings.

We have found that our horses are almost immune to skin diseases, distemper, and other contagious diseases after they have been wintered in South Carolina and brought to the tracks where these ailments are taking their toll. You have observed how quickly we can cure these various ailments in young horses. We believe that the blood is so cleansed by the action of iodine from your feeds and water, that all common infections are removed, and the system so toned up that it is in shape to fight and ward off anything except direct infection through an open wound. A few years ago a good trainer was one who could bring his horses to the races well fed and bulging with muscle. But the make-up of these muscles, and the contents of the bloodstream feeding them, is the determining factor in having a really fit and ready horse.

In appreciation of the good you have done our horses, and the things we have learned from your efforts, we trust that you will find time this coming season to again spend considerable time at the fair grounds, and conduct further experiments on our stock.

In order to learn whether instinct played a part in leading dairy cows to food rich in iodine, the owner of a mixed herd of 54 cows which I had previously studied built a special feeding station for me at the end of the lane leading from the barnyard. The station was divided into four compartments, roofed over to protect them from rain.

In one compartment was placed a feeding supplement, nationally advertised, which contained iodine and other minerals in inorganic form. The second compartment was supplied with bone meal, the third compartment with a feeding supplement made of ocean kelp, in which all the minerals are in organic form. The fourth compartment contained salt.

We stood nearby to observe what happened when the cows passed this feeding station for the first time.

Each cow sniffed at each compartment. They passed by without touching the feeding supplement made of inorganic minerals. A few took some of the bone meal, and a few some of the salt. But what they really converged on was the kelp, which as has been said contains more iodine than anything else that grows. As fast as we could fill up the compartment, they would clean it out. This settled the point for us: cows like iodine and in organic, which is to say natural, form.

Subsequently I offered kelp to two registered Jersey bulls in the barn. They took it quickly and teased for more.

One of my friends raises hunting dogs as a hobby. The dogs are Brittany spaniels. When they have been trained to hunt, he sells them.

Being impressed by the favorable effects of apple cider vinegar on his own health and body endurance, he asked me if it would be all right to try giving the vinegar to his dogs. He thought they tired too easily when hunting. We decided on the following method. When the dogs were not hunting, one tablespoonful of apple cider vinegar would be added to the ration of each dog once a day. When they were hunting, there would be a tablespoonful added twice a day. After following this method for three years at these kennels, the following conclusions were reached:

If a hunting dog has (1) one tablespoonful of apple cider vinegar added to his ration once a day during the off-hunting season; (2), one tablespoonful added to his ration twice a day when used for hunting; (3) one tablespoonful added to his drinking water while hunting, whenever he is given a drink; (4) one tablespoonful of undiluted vinegar when the dog is thirsty and no drinking water is available, the following results were noted:

1. A dog receiving the apple cider vinegar will not tire easily. The average dog that has not received it is good for three to four hours of hunting a day. A dog receiving it will hunt eight to ten hours steady during the day. Apple cider vinegar clearly increases the hunting dog's endurance.

2. A dog receiving the apple cider vinegar will be able to point and retrieve every bird for as many as four hunters hunting at the same time.

3. A dog receiving the vinegar will not show shortness of breath at any time while hunting.

4. A dog receiving the vinegar will maintain a good appetite and eat every meal while being used for hunting.

5. A dog receiving the vinegar will not lose weight while hunting.

Having now traced the use of iodine to increase the speed and endurance of race horses and the endurance of hunting dogs, let us adapt what we have learned to the health side of the daily life of a business executive.

On rising in the morning he will drink a glass of water while dressing into which one or two teaspoonfuls of apple cider vinegar has been mixed. What may he expect to accomplish by doing this?

The knowledge that acids thin body fluids has been brought over from the days when blood-letting was a common form of treatment. We have found in the barn that the milk of a normal cow is weakly acid. When the reaction of the milk changes to alkaline, the milk becomes soup-thick. This thickness will disappear and the milk will return to its normal watery character, however, if and when the cow is given four ounces of apple cider vinegar and four ounces of water by mouth from a bottle, night and morning.

There are other ways of observing this principle in action but this is sufficient here. The point is, no busy executive wants his blood to be on the thick side, like soup; he understands that it should be thin, in order to circulate easily throughout the body, making easy work for his heart as it pumps blood with each beat.

At breakfast this man omits wheat foods, wheat cereals, white sugar, and citrus fruits and fruit juices because in the majority of people these foods change the normal acid reaction of the urine to alkaline. The alkalinity is a signal that the blood is thicker than it should be, that it is not easily circulated and requires more heart effort to pump it. Therefore this man replaces these unwise foods with rye and corn foods and cereals. Instead of white sugar he uses honey. In place of citrus foods and citrus juices he takes the contents of a bottle of fruit sold at the grocery store under the name

Junior Foods. Or, if he chooses, he may take apple, grape, or cranberry juice.

At lunchtime he takes two teaspoonfuls of apple cider vinegar and two teaspoonfuls of honey in a glass of water. In this way he obtains acid taken up from the soil by fruit, berries, edible leaves, and roots, and the energy from the sun which exists in honey. This is a prime pick-up drink. He may take it before, during, or after lunch. A vinegar made from the whole crushed apple is best for the purpose, such as those sold under the brand names Heinz or Sterling.

When a person is organizing his body for a day of dynamic action, the organization shifts the urine reaction from the normal, or acid, to the alkaline. It is not advisable, therefore, to eat foods at the morning meal which will, so to speak, duplicate the shift. For this reason the wheat foods, white sugar, and citrus fruits and their juices are omitted, so that at the end of the day he will return home with less mental and physical fatigue.

At the evening meal he will also take the two teaspoonfuls of honey and two teaspoonfuls of apple cider vinegar in a glass of water. He may like to take it before the meal, as a cocktail, or during the meal.

It is beneficial also to start the meal with a leafy green salad, to get the benefit of the acid from the soil and the energy from the sun stored up in the leaves.

If the day has been one of overwork and anxiety, turn to fish or other seafood, for that will supply the iodine and potassium that will calm down the nervous system.

Try to have such muscle meats as beef, lamb, or pork only twice a week, and then on days when you have a light schedule, because muscle meat organizes your body on a combat basis, which you do not want from food. Try to bear in mind that the internal organs of an animal, such as the liver, represent the animal storehouse against the time of need. It will be well for you to have liver or liverwurst once a week. Gradually, by following the foregoing plan, you can make changes in your daily food selection so that the intake will counterbalance your heavy expenditure of strength and energy.

Supposing you do follow the suggestions outlined above and yet find that some weeks the pressures of your private and your business life are causing you to lose the ability to bounce back. Then you should add a drop of Lugol's solution of iodine to your glass of apple or grape juice at breakfast, or you may take it in the mixture of apple cider vinegar and water. The point is that the potassium in the solution blocks off the body mechanism that organizes for aggressive action, releasing its hold on the body when opportunity for rest and relaxation arises. The iodine swings into action the body mechanism which organizes the body for peace and quiet and the building up and storing of body reserves. When working under pressure, include the Lugol's solution dose each day until the period of pressure passes. If it should happen that your body becomes saturated with iodine, you will find that there is an increase of moisture in the nose. If this occurs, omit the iodine until the nose is normal.

As you study yourself you will soon learn to tell when you need iodine. When a night's sleep does not bring you to the beginning of the new day with the energy you are accustomed to have, you will begin to think of iodine. If you learn how to use it, it will restore the capacity to bounce back and sustain your well-being.

CHAPTER XII

Castor Oil and Corn Oil

ONE CANNOT STUDY Vermont folk medicine many years without becoming interested in castor oil for the versatile place it occupies in therapeutic measures. I am not now referring to its classic cathartic action, but rather to its local action on the skin, and tissues beneath the skin.

My first awareness of external uses of castor oil came when a successful rural general practitioner told me that he used castor oil for removal of warts. I began to collect various uses, among them the following:

1. The method of dealing with warts is to apply the oil night and morning to the wart, rubbing it 20 times or so, to work the oil well into the excrescence.

2. Castor oil, I learned, is a favorite application for an ulcer on the body.

3. Among elderly native Vermont women in connection with the various necessities of midwifery, it was common knowledge that castor oil was applied to the navel of a newborn infant if for any reason it showed difficulty in healing.

4. Castor oil is applied to the breasts to increase the flow of milk.

5. If the eye develops redness and irritation, one drop of castor oil dropped in the eye makes it more comfortable and relieves irritation.

6. If little children fail to show a proper growth and development of the hair on the head, castor oil should be applied to the

head twice a week at bedtime. The oil is rubbed thoroughly into the scalp, is allowed to remain overnight, and in the morning removed by a shampoo. By using the oil twice a week until a satisfactory change in the hair is established, the health of the hair can be maintained by applying this treatment once in two weeks or once a month.

7. Castor oil, applied to the eyelashes at bedtime three times a week, will thicken them and make them grow longer. The same treatment applies to eyebrow growth.

8. Castor oil is used in the eyes of hunting dogs to clear up an eye condition produced by running through grass.

9. In a chest cold or bronchitis, a mixture of two tablespoonfuls of castor oil and one tablespoonful of spirits of turpentine is applied to the chest. First the castor oil is warmed, then the spirits of turpentine added. The mixture is rubbed into the chest a little, then the chest covered with a warm cloth. If the difficulty is mild, the mixture is applied at bedtime; if it is severe, application should be made three times a day.

10. In many farm homes a bottle of castor oil is always kept on hand. And people who know the ways of folk medicine are quick to apply castor oil with a feather to any cut, abrasion, or sore on the body.

11. When hemorrhoids come outside of the anal ring, castor oil will soften them so that they may be reversed.

12. Twice a week, or more often if the feet are working overtime, the feet may be rubbed down at bedtime with castor oil. Cotton socks are slipped on and the oil left on overnight. In the morning the skin is like velvet, and generally all the tired, sore feeling will have disappeared. In the same way castor oil can be used night and morning to soften corns and calluses and remove the soreness. Castor oil is considered a specific remedy for soft corns.

Having informed myself as to these various uses of castor oil in Vermont folk medicine, I began trying them out, with the following results.

A patient, who was sixty-four years old and a lawyer and who had a wart on the edge of his right nostril, applied castor oil to it night and morning, working the oil well into the wart with his finger. At the end of three weeks the wart had disappeared.

While adjusting the eyeglasses of a patient sixty-two years old, I noticed that she had a papilloma 3x3x3mm at the outer end of her left eyebrow. This had a smooth surface and appeared like a skin-colored miniature grape. I asked how long it had been there, and she said three months. I suggested that at each mealtime she apply castor oil to the papilloma and let me know the result. At the end of six weeks it had disappeared to the degree that I would never have known it had been there.

Another woman, forty-nine years of age, had a papilloma on the right cheek which she told me had been present for at least ten years, perhaps even longer. It was annoying to her because when she dried her face, the towel was apt to catch on the papilloma. I measured it and found it to be 6x6 millimeters, and 5 millimeters high. At the end of two weeks of using the castor oil as prescribed in the other cases, its size had lessened so that it no longer caught on the towel when she dried her face. At the end of one month it was measured again and the size had decreased to 4x4 millimeters, and 3 millimeters high.

A young married woman thirty years of age came to Vermont with her three children to spend the summer with her father, who had retired and returned to Vermont to live. While seeing her father I observed that she had a brown mole, in the middle of her right cheek, about the size of her little fingernail. It was so brown that it showed through her make-up. I told her I thought castor oil might influence the mole favorably, if she cared to try it. Telling me that it had been there ever since she could remember, she accepted my suggestion. Each evening when she removed her make-up she thoroughly rubbed in the castor oil, wiping off the excess with a tissue as she was about to get into bed. At the end of one week she noticed that the color of the mole had begun to fade. By the end of three weeks the brown had completely disappeared. I could see a smooth place where the mole had been, but its color was that of the surrounding skin.

After success with moles, I became interested in the problem of the brown "liver spots," so called, which appear on the face and hands of the aging. I wondered whether they would be favorably influenced by castor oil. I found a patient who had about a dozen such brown spots on the back of each hand and I suggested that castor oil be applied night and morning, rubbing it well into the skin. The patient was glad to try it, for he wanted to get rid of the spots.

By the end of one month they had all disappeared; had I not seen them, I would never have known they had been there.

Because all corn products are accepted very well by natives of the Vermont environment, I extended my studies in applications of oil to possible uses of vegetable oils made from the hearts of full-ripened corn kernels. While originally produced for cooking purposes, I was to find that corn oil has valuable medicinal qualities as well. Among its advantages it is easily obtainable, not expensive, and is pleasant to take, being almost tasteless.

Corn oils are a good source of acid. The complete analysis of one of them, Mazola Oil, with each acid calculated on a basis of total fat, is as follows:

	Per cent
Linolenic Acid	1.85
Linoleic Acid	38.24
Oleic Acid	42.78
Palmitric Acid	7.56
Stearic Acid	4.82
Arachidic Acid	.22
Lignoceric Acid	Trace

The following observations have been made in prescribing corn oil:

When added to treatment previously indicated, one table-spoonful of corn oil at one or all three meals each day has been helpful in hay fever, asthma, and migraine, because it helps in keeping the urine reaction on the acid side. Corn oil is of value in shifting the body chemistry from alkaline to acid.

These further results have been noted:

If the margins of the eyelids are scaly and granulated, one tablespoonful of corn oil by mouth at breakfast, and again at the evening meal, will, within one month's time, generally cure the condition. If there is present on the body one or more patches of dry, scaly eczema, the same treatment will often cause the scaliness to disappear in from one to two months. Useful in cleansing an area of eczema, it will remove scales when present, leaving the skin soft and pliable.

One tablespoonful of corn oil at one or all three meals each day has been very helpful in controlling angioneurotic edema, which is characterized by a sudden swelling of one of the lips, the side of the face, or a place on the forehead. When such swelling does occur, the corn oil taken by mouth will generally cause it to disappear.

I have learned from patients also that the treatment is beneficial in disturbances of the hair and scalp. Taken twice a day by mouth, if hair is lifeless and difficult to handle with brush and comb, corn oil taken internally at breakfast and evening will, within one to two months' time, restore gloss to the hair and make it easy to arrange. The treatment will generally cure dandruff in one to two months' time. And the oil makes a valuable regular shampoo. I give the following directions to patients for this purpose: Warm the oil and massage it thoroughly into the scalp. Wrap a towel, wrung out of hot water, about the head. Repeat the hot-towel application five or six times. Now shampoo with a mild soap. The result will be hair so glossy that it shines. I have had mothers drop into my office just to show me how fine and soft their children's hair was after a corn oil shampoo; each hair seemed to stand up to be counted, shining as though it had been varnished.

All in all I have become thoroughly convinced by experience that there are sound underlying reasons for the uses made of oils in Vermont folk medicine. They remind us again that all folk medicine has grown out of the ready availability of natural preventive and curative substances. Oils are to be found in plants on every side. If we stop only long enough to remind ourselves that Nature is all-wise, we do not need to ask ourselves, "Will this work?" Nature built in its guarantees.

CHAPTER XIII

Medical Reasoning Behind
Vermont Folk Medicine

SOME YEARS AGO a woman patient advanced in years brought me in a book published in 1824. She was a maiden lady. "I'm the last of the family, so there'll be no more use for this when I'm gone, and I would like you to have it." The title of the book is *The American Botanist and Family Physician.* The book concerns itself with the medical virtues of the mineral, animal, and vegetable elements in Nature and their uses in the practice of physical medicine and surgery.

Looking back over my studies in and experiments with Vermont folk medicine, I ask myself, What are its approaches in solving the medical problems presented in human individuals?

Because of the weather variability, which is an important characteristic of Vermont, the first thing Vermont folk medicine checks when sickness is present is the weather impact. When there is a drop in the outdoor temperature the blood reaction immediately becomes more alkaline, the adrenal glands more active, blood pressure rises, and, as the blood becomes more alkaline, tissue chemistry is altered. Conversely, when the outdoor temperature rises for a few days the blood becomes less alkaline, activity of the adrenal glands

153

decreases, blood pressure goes down, and tissue chemistry alters in relation to prevailing conditions.

How does Vermont folk medicine teach that the body can be protected against frequent and taxing weather changes? Basically by maintaining the body reaction acid, instead of alkaline. How can this be accomplished? By a daily intake of acid, the amount depending on the coldness of the weather. What is an ideal form of acid intake? Apple cider vinegar which, utilizing the whole apple, represents a pure form of ideal elements. How is it taken? One or more tea-spoonfuls of apple cider vinegar in a glass of water, one or two times a day.

Having checked the weather impact, Vermont folk medi-cine turns next to the impact of environment. Vermont as a state is iodine-poor. Its topsoil does not have as much potassium as could be desired from the health standpoint of those who live close to the land. Potassium is to the nervous system what calcium is to bone. Potassium deficiency can be compensated by adding a drop of Lugol's solution to the daily intake of apple cider vinegar; Lugol's solution is a 5% elemental iodine dissolved in a 10% solution of potas-sium iodide. This meets the body's need for iodine and potassium.

An example of environmental impact upon the body is a ringing, buzzing, hissing or other sensation of noise in one or both ears. Such a disagreeable condition can be overcome by the treatment indicated above.

"Environmental factors" is no mere phrase. Environmental factors may be described as resembling the instruments of a symphony orchestra. Each instrument in itself makes music, but each music has its own sound. All the instruments make music by playing notes. In the well-being of the body each factor produces its own clinical results. As with the instru-ments in symphonic music, it is the interaction of environ-mental factors, producing their clinical results by means of their action in the mechanism of the body, that organizes the body "music," for good or ill.

When Vermont folk medicine has checked both weather and environmental impact, it turns to the impact of food on the body. It holds that we build and rebuild our "human house" by means of the food we eat, the liquid we drink, the air we breathe. As the racial strain dominant in the individual is an important factor, it is estimated and, as far as possible to do so, the individual is returned to his racial diet. During the passing centuries the race he represents has worked out by the trial and error method the daily food intake best suited to it; it, in turn, has developed a type of body that will work best on that racial diet.

When weather, environmental and food impacts on the body have been checked Vermont folk medicine turns its attention next to the immemorial duel between the body cell and the harmful microorganisms. It is difficult, of course, to cooperate with Nature unless we know what her health program is. When we know that harmful microorganisms grow on an alkaline soil, and that Nature has liberally surrounded us with acids in the form of fruits, berries, edible roots and edible leaves, we can better appreciate the need of following Nature's advice, by taking in each day enough acid to prevent body tissues from becoming alkaline soil congenial to the growth of pathogenic microorganisms.

We are all pretty much alike in that we wish for continuous good health and to have the energy and endurance which will make enjoyably productive both our work and play. I can assure you that if you follow the pathway outlined, you will come to the December of your life with good digestion, good eyesight, good hearing, good mental and physical vigor.

We are prone to believe we know a great deal about the body and how to keep it in trim. In the relative sense, this is true. But we are far from knowing all we might. For me it has required many years of study to understand Vermont folk medicine and the medical reasoning upon which it proceeds. In one sense it might be called an old-fashioned medicine. Certainly it has existed a long time in daily practice. It is primarily preventive; its roots are far back in primitive living when people and animals, constantly on the move, simply did not have time to be sick.

Civilization, with its stresses and strains, has brought many new variations of diseases and sickness, yet the underlying principles of Vermont folk medicine continue to be a constant means of pushing back horizons of knowledge about them. Civilization has brought no new physiological and biochemical laws and has not successfully amended any of the old ones. Nature saw to it all at the outset, by creating the body ideally, in balance. Sickness is the posing of a problem in restoring the balance when it has knowingly or unknowingly been interfered with. Sickness is the road sign telling us that we have tried to wander cross-lots, off the main road Nature laid out for us.

Having been trained in the approaches and methods of organized medicine, I became very curious as to that considerable body of knowledge and practice called Vermont folk medicine. I set myself certain goals of study and research. In many ways no environment for studying and testing folk medicine could be more stern than the environment of Vermont. I am of the opinion that measures which work well under the rigors of Vermont conditions may be expected to work even more easily where climatic conditions are less harsh and capricious.

I have come to the end of the studies and research I laid out to do. Now you might say I'm sitting back—still interested in how it works out.

APPENDIX A

FURTHER STUDIES MADE ON ANIMALS

Chickens receiving apple cider vinegar in their drinking water grow faster, feather out quicker, are hardier, and are much larger. At the end of three weeks all chickens were fully feathered and tails were starting to grow. They develop more meat on their bony frame; the additional meat is lean meat; the chickens are plump when cooked.

I wrote a doctor friend who as a hobby raises turkeys about my experience in adding apple cider vinegar to the drinking water of chickens. He became interested and decided to add the vinegar to the drinking water of his turkeys. Later he reported to me the following observations: When these turkeys were slaughtered and served as food the meat was found to be unusually tender. When the bones of a newly slaughtered turkey were broken, it was found that the bone marrow showed an increased redness, indicating a better formation of red blood cells needed by the blood.

Mink are predatory animals and are therefore meat eaters. In the mink herd I studied, the animals are fed once a day. This herd numbered 1200 females and 300 males. They are mated each year during the month of March. As a result of this mating, 3500 little mink are born each year. They grow to adult size in three months and are pelted in November and December, and the pelts are marketed.

The following observations have been made on mink. A mink will accept 11 per cent protein in its ration. At one time the protein content of the ration for all the mink was raised to 20 per cent. When this happened, mink began to die. At autopsy these mink showed a bladder full of stones. These stones were sent to a laboratory for analysis. The report stated that they were urate stones. Forty mink died from the stones which the laboratory said were due to too much protein in the ration. When the protein in the ration was lowered back to 11 per cent, no mink were lost from bladder stones. This observation suggests that a relation exists between a high protein intake and stone formation in the kidneys and bladder in human individuals.

Mink have a severe form of dizziness often referred to as Ménière's syndrome. They will stagger and walk around in circles, and later will whirl in circles, grabbing the tips of their tails and biting them in an effort, by hanging on to them, to steady themselves. If this dizziness continues, they continue biting their tails as they whirl until in time they have chewed down the whole length of a 10-inch tail. When this happens the male mink is valueless because, in breeding a female, he sets himself, bracing his body by his tail to maintain the mating position. The mink literature I have read states positively that staggering, walking around in circles, and whirling are due to too much protein in the ration. I learned also that mink in the wild state get the acid they need by eating berries and leaves which are acid in reaction.

I suggested to the owner of the mink herd I studied that one-fourth of a teaspoonful of apple cider vinegar be added to the ration for each mink showing this tendency to staggering gait, whirling, and tail chewing. The difficulty seems to be most common in the pastel shades of mink. Also these pastel-shade mink carry their heads on one side, with one ear higher than the other. As far as I know there is no explanation of this habit.

Some of the pastel mink in the herd were sold for mating purposes. The new owners did not add the apple cider vinegar to the ration, with the result that the difficulties of staggering gait and so on returned. This strengthens the indication that an acid must be taken with animal protein food, in order to avoid imbalances in the body.

During my study of a herd of goats, the herd developed a cobalt deficiency. Cobalt is a trace mineral. I never realized before the extent to which a body can be wrecked by the deficiency of just one trace mineral, even when the amount needed is so little as to be passed by almost unnoticed. These observations will illustrate how important trace minerals are to the proper performance of the body processes:

1. During the month of February one of the female goats in this herd began to show scales on her body. I was asked what was wrong. I did not know.

2. Goats in the herd began to be fussy in their eating. One day they would eat well, the next day they would show loss of appetite, only to regain appetite the following day.

3. Their coat of hair changed. It lost its luster and began to fall out. Hair also became brittle.

4. Instead of starting a pregnancy after one serving by a buck as had been the custom in this herd, it required three different breedings before a goat started a pregnancy.

Many other perplexing manifestations appeared. In all, 17 goats died, presenting one picture or another of unexpected difficulty.

The local veterinary could not make out a diagnosis. A nutrition specialist was contacted who was employed by a wholesale company preparing foods for market for the feeding of livestock. He came to the goat farm and made a diagnosis of cobalt deficiency.

Dr. Wallter, a veterinary on the teaching staff of the Department of Agriculture, University of Vermont, was also contacted. He confirmed the diagnosis of cobalt deficiency as being responsible for the physical condition of goats in the herd.

It requires four years of a lack of cobalt in the food of goats before symptoms of the deficiency become evident. From this observation one surmises that, in human individuals, a mineral deficiency must be present for some time before symptoms arise that lead an individual to consult a physician. When a cobalt deficiency is present, an animal is very susceptible to pneumonia and to infections of all kinds.

One fourth of an ounce of cobalt to a ton of hay is all that is necessary to avoid a cobalt deficiency. With the herd of goats, by trial and error it was learned that the treatment dose of a solution made by adding one ounce of cobalt sulphate crystals, commercial grade, and thoroughly dissolving it in one gallon of water, was one teaspoonful twice a day for ten days, then once a day as the condition of the goat showed its need. It was fed once a day for 13 weeks. At the end of that time the cobalt was discontinued because the goats began to lose weight and it was thought they might have reached the toxic level for cobalt. If while receiving cobalt a goat lost its appetite, it was given $\frac{1}{4}$ to $\frac{1}{3}$ cup of granulated sugar twice daily. This sugar restored the appetite in 24 hours.

Cobalt is truly a trace element, as are boron, magnesium, copper, iron, and iodine. The exact work of these trace elements in plant, animal, and human nutrition is not easy to explain. We understand the need in both animals and humans for nitrogen, potash, phosphate, water, and sunshine. Perhaps it is easiest to say that these trace minerals act as catalysts that enable the plant, animal, or human being to make more perfect use of the more common food elements.

When I decided to study some dairy herds with special reference to proteins, I went to a friend, a bacteriologist at the Barre Cooperative Creamery, and asked him to suggest herds for me to study. The first he suggested was the Ernest Bisson herd of 54 cows. This was a mixed herd including various breeds of cattle. The herd replacements were not raised but were purchased from cattle dealers and farmers. Calves when born in this herd were sold to cattle dealers. My bacteriological friend told me that Ernest Bisson made more milk per cow than any other of the 250 farmers that brought milk to the creamery. He worked his herd hard. In addition to making the most milk per cow, he also had more herd troubles than any other farmer bringing milk to the creamery. The creamery was constantly alerted for the appearance of streptococci in milk from this herd.

A second herd he suggested was a herd of 45 registered Jersey cows. The young woman in charge of the herd was a graduate of a Midwest agricultural college and was considered an outstanding herdswoman in Vermont. Her cattle were consistent prize winners at fairs and Jersey cattle shows. Emphasis in this herd is on breeding and the raising of young cattle to be sold as a source of income.

In addition to the above two herds, my brother-in-law in southern Vermont had an outstanding herd of 50 prize-winning Holsteins, which I visited from time to time.

Ernest Bisson welcomed me in discussions of herds and the "protein problem." He had two brothers who were successful medical men. He had asked them for advice as to how he might solve herd problems but they had not been able to give the help he desired. He had turned to the Agriculture Department of the University of Vermont for help with the problem of mastitis in a cow's udder, but there was mastitis in the college herd too and they had not found out how to solve it. He was told that mastitis in the cow's udder was due to an infection which they did not know how to control.

I asked him to list his herd problems so that I might familiarize myself with them. I wrote them down as follows:

1. Mastitis, both acute and chronic. At the time of my visit seven cows were marked for slaughter for beef because of the presence of chronic mastitis, with streptococci present in the milk from one or more quarters of the udder.

2. Inability to start a pregnancy in 20 cows out of the total herd number of 54. Some had not started a pregnancy for as long as one year. This failure to start a pregnancy disrupted Bisson's breeding program so that he could not plan the lactation periods of the cows in his herd.

3. Brucellosis in his herd. The presence of abortions due to brucellosis meant the loss of calves to serve as herd replacements. Calves that were born were weak and generally died within two weeks. This made it impossible for him to raise young stock to serve as herd replacements, and the abortions spoiled the lactation period of the mother cow.

4. Poor potency in the herd bulls made repeated breedings necessary before a pregnancy could be started.

5. Loss of appetite in cows.

6. Prolonged labor in cows.

7. Because of being unable to raise his herd replacements, he had to purchase them from near-by farmers and cattle dealers. This meant buying problem cows, because farmers do not sell their best cows.

8. Arthritis in some cows, making it difficult for them to lie down and get up.

9. Increased susceptibility of herd cows to colds.

10. Influenza in herd cows during the winter months.

11. Leg paralysis of some of herd cows, commonly referred to as "milk fever," following the births of their calves.

12. Constipation in herd cows.

This was quite a list of herd troubles and the list represented quite a challenge in solution.

I next asked Miss Stone, who had charge of the herd of 45 registered Jersey cows, to list her herd problems, so that at the beginning of my study I might have something definite to work on. She listed them as follows:

1. Abortions in the herd, lessening the number of young cattle that could be offered for sale.

2. Lack of uniform size in calves when born.

3. Weakness of calves when born.

4. Calves do not have the uniform markings of the mother cow or the bull, which mean so much when the calf is later offered for sale as a herd replacement.

5. Difficulty in breeding cows, which do not start a pregnancy after the first breeding.

Having recorded the list of troubles in the two herds, I purchased an apparatus which would receive leaves, flowers, and grass at one end and, by the turning of a crank, yield juice. I also laid in a supply of Squibb's Nitrazine Paper because it has a wide reaction range, from pH 4.5 on the acid side, to pH 7.5 on the alkaline side. With the juicing machine, the bottle of Nitrazine Paper, a note book, a pail of water, and a cup to wash out the juice-extracting apparatus after each extraction, I started following these two herds on pasture during the warmer months of the year. By following them many hours, I learned many things about nutrition.

The Ernest Bisson farm was a hillside farm with very few trees or bushes in the pastures. The farm where the 45 Jerseys were kept was a valley farm with a small river running through it. Every pasture on this farm contained trees and bushes.

I felt that the contrast between the two farms was fortunate as a study factor.

I first followed the herd on the hillside farm. When I juiced what this herd selected for eating, I found it was always acid in reaction. When I juiced what they passed by, refusing to eat, I found it was always alkaline in reaction. Where there had been cow droppings in the pasture the grass growing on the spot was taller and darker green. This made the grass attractive in size and color. But the cows did not eat this grass; they avoided the spots carefully. When I tested the juice from the grass growing in these manure spots, the juice always tested alkaline in reaction. The instinctive refusal of these dairy cows to eat alkaline-reaction grass suggested that the dairy cow is by nature a good chemist and that here she was trying to bring about a balanced chemistry in her body. Clearly she was also a good soil chemist and my time would not be wasted by going to school to her.

Next I went to the farm where I could observe the registered Jerseys on pasture. I was impressed at once with their fondness for the leaves available to them in the different verdure of these pastures. I took a sampling of the leaves and on juicing them found them acid in reaction. I also observed that as a rule the cows preferred to eat where the growth was most recent.

I discussed this fondness for leaves with Miss Stone, the herdswoman in charge. She confirmed the preference and added that she had never received a mastitis warning from the creamery to which the herd milk was sent.

Miss Stone was very much interested in my study of the herd and said she would try to set up some experiments for me which might be fruitful. One day she telephoned to say that she was about to turn the herd into pasture where kale was in blossom; if I wished, she would do so when I could be present.

When the herd of 45 cows entered this field the first thing I noted was that they ate all the kale blossoms before eating any other vegetation growing in the field. I tested the juice of the kale blossoms and it was acid in reaction.

Another day Miss Stone telephoned me that she was about to turn the herd into a field of second-growth clover which could not be harvested because of lack of time.

Around the edge of this field chokecherry trees had seeded themselves in years past and had reached full growth. When turned into this field the cows never touched the clover but went at once to the chokecherry trees, eating the leaves on them all the way up, even standing on their hind legs to reach the higher ones. The cows had avoided the alkaline-reacting clover in favor of the acid-reacting chokecherry leaves.

At another time this herd was turned into a field where potatoes had been grown and harvested. A few potatoes had been missed and these the cows dug up with their hoofs; when they had finished I believe they had not missed one. Here again was the acid reaction, in the potatoes.

I asked Miss Stone whether she would be willing to fertilize part of one of the pastures with manure and, as soon as vegetation had had time to appear, turn the young cattle into the field to see whether, guided by instinct, they would avoid the manured portion or would accept vegetation growing there.

Subsequently sixteen head of young cattle were turned into a pasture where about one fourth of the field had been fertilized with cow manure the previous fall. The manure had been under the barn for one year. The grass in this section of field was much greener and taller than the grass in the rest of the pasture. The dividing line between the fertilized and unfertilized portions of the field was easily seen. The young cattle ranged in age from six months to one year.

Of the sixteen head only two grazed in the manure-fertilized area of the field. They were aged about six months. Even while I stood watching them, they left this fertilized section and went to graze that part of the pasture not thus fertilized.

I had occasion at this same dairy farm to see a different illustration of the chemical sagacity of cows. There was one cow here which was twenty years old; for sentimental reasons it was given a place in the barn. The aged cow was called Bobby, and she had the run of the farm. I spent considerable time following her as she roamed about, as I wanted to learn her eating habits. She was very fond of elm leaves and ate them in preference to all other leaves. I know little about the composition of elm leaves except that they are acid in reaction. I have observed here in Vermont that, when a farmer going after cows early in the morning discovers that he is hungry, he eats one or two elm leaves if they are available; it does away with the hunger sensation, and his appetite is satisfied.

It was customary to tie Bobby loosely in the barn, so that it would be easier for her to get up and down. One day she broke loose. Making for the feed car, she tried to get into the apple cider vinegar pail kept there. Miss Stone heard the rattling of the pail and went to investigate. In order to see just what old Bobby would do, Miss Stone put the vinegar pail on the floor of the car. Bobby proceeded to lap up about a pint of the vinegar and then, evidently satisfied, turned away. This suggested to us that the aging animal body needs acid too, and knows it.

A plate count of the milk delivered by each creamery supplier is made each week. Makers of ordinary milk are allowed 400,000 bacteria in each cubic centimeter of unpasteurized milk and 20,000 bacteria in each cubic centimeter of pasteurized milk.

However, the two herds I studied at this time made Grade A milk, which requires higher standards. The milk from one herd was sent to Massachusetts, milk from the other to Rhode Island. Creamery suppliers of Grade A milk are allowed a 50,000 unpasteurized-milk bacteria plate count, and a 5000 pasteurized-milk bacteria plate count in each cubic centimeter of milk. When a supplier has a high bacteria count it may be due to unclean milking utensils or trouble in a cow, he is given two weeks in which to get it cleared up.

A plate count is made in the following way:

Take 1 cubic centimeter of milk to be tested. To this add 99 cubic centimeters of sterile water. Put 1 cubic centimeter of the above mixture in a petri dish. Add to the 1 cubic centimeter of the above mixture 10 cubic centimeters of sterile culture media. Incubate at 92F for 48 hours. Each group of bacteria will make a colony that can be seen with the naked eye. Count colonies of bacteria in whole petri dish, and multiply by 100 to give number of bacteria in 1 cubic centimeter of milk. Colonies of bacteria may be counted with low microscope magnification.

On receipt of copies of two letters congratulating each herd owner on the low bacteria count of the milk from his herd, I began to experiment further and learned that, when the apple cider vinegar was omitted, the bacteria count of the milk went up; when the herd received its vinegar quota each day, the bacteria count of the milk went down. In this connection the following figures are of interest:

PLATE COUNT REPORTS FROM MIXED HERD OF 54 COWS

Grade A Unpasteurized Milk Allowed 50,000 bacteria for each cubic centimeter 1944		Grade A Pasteurized Milk Allowed 5,000 bacteria for each cubic centimeter 1944
April 12	20,000	800
April 28	3,500	1,000
May 13	30,000	500
May 18	30,000	800
May 25	3,000	600
May 30	10,000	800
June 14	48,000	2,300
June 21	40,000	1,200
June 29	22,000	600

At the end of five years of study and close observation of this herd of 54 dairy cows, in winter quarters in the barn during the colder months, on pasture through the warmer months, my farmer friend and I reviewed the list of original herd troubles, to learn what progress had been made in our going to school to the cows, and to try to interpret and put into further regular practice what they had taught us. The following had resulted from measures used:

1. Not a cow had been slaughtered for two years because of the presence of mastitis in the udder. Chronic mastitis was no longer in his herd.

2. As for cows not starting a pregnancy, during the five years his herd had increased to 70 cows because of successful control of mastitis. Out of 70 cows only eight had failed during the past year to start a pregnancy. Of the original 20 that failed to start a pregnancy when I began to study the herd, all 20 started a pregnancy within four months' time.

3. As for brucellosis, in his herd this condition remained to be solved. Some progress had, however, been made. The abortions were fewer, only three cows aborting during the past year. Too the abortion was now postponed until the last month of pregnancy. And cows that did abort no longer lost their lactation period, but started it as they would have if the calf went to full term pregnancy.

4. There had been no trouble in maintaining the potency of bulls in the herd.

5. There was no longer loss of appetite present in cows.

6. Prolonged labor in giving birth to calves had disappeared; cows now had a short, normal labor. If it happened that a placenta retained by a cow after giving birth to a calf, it was generally delivered in four days. While the placenta was being retained, there was no odor or discharge, as had been the case in the past.

7. No weak, fussy calves were being born.

8. Only one cow in the herd had developed arthritis, and this soon cleared up.

9. Disappearance of head colds in cows.

10. No influenza and no pneumonia.

11. No milk fever with leg paralysis, when cows give birth to their calf.

12. No constipation in cows. If diarrhea does appear, it is promptly made to disappear.

In like manner I went over her original herd troubles with Miss Stone. We recorded the following results from measures used:

1. Abortions in the herd had been stopped.

2. Calves were no longer born undersized.

3. When born calves were strong and rugged, with strong legs and much hair on the body. They were up on their feet within five minutes of birth and nursing at the cows' udders before they were a half hour old.

4. Calves when born were now uniform in markings. They had intelligence. It was no longer necessary to teach them to drink from a pail, as they seemed to have brought the knowledge across from the mother.

5. Breeding troubles in the herd had disappeared, and repeated breeding of cows was no longer a problem.

It is more widely recognized by dairymen now that too much protein may be a source of udder trouble. A farmer may be feeding a certain per cent of protein in his herd ration which seems to work well with the herd. Suddenly he runs into some early-cut hay that is rich in protein. The protein in the ration and in the early-cut hay now adds up to too much protein, with the result that udder trouble appears in some of the cows.

There is a valuable comparison between the daily intake for cows and for human diet. A cow receiving apple cider vinegar on her ration twice a day will eat less hay and grain. A person who adds a teaspoonful or two of the vinegar to a glass of water and consumes it during a meal will be satisfied with less food. This meets Nature's original plans, which included giving a place to a natural acid intake in the whole diet.

I then turned to a book, *The Jersey*, published by the American Jersey Cattle Club which gives the history of the Jersey cow and her background on the Island of Jersey. I was particularly interested in the soil on the island and the fertilizers used.

It seems that the Jersey soils all have an acid tendency. There is neither limestone nor chalk on the island. Fertilizing is with seaweed washed up on shore after ocean storms. The farmers gather the seaweed from the beaches at low tide. Besides humus and potassium, seaweed adds sodium and iodine to the soil, and also the rest of the 46 minerals contained in seaweed.

Soon after reading this book I heard of a Jersey herd in which each cow had been imported from the Island of Jersey. I sought an opportunity to visit the herd and was at once impressed with the animals' length of body. I had never seen such long-bodied Jersey cows. The herd bull, at the time of his importation champion of the island bulls, also had a body that was unusually long. To me this reflected the potassium content of the seaweed used to fertilize the land. And it confirmed that in their ancestral island Jerseys find the acid soil, potassium, iodine, and other needed minerals sought by Jersey cows in Vermont.

I now asked the late Professor George W. Cavanaugh, Professor of Agricultural Chemistry at Cornell University, where the prize-winning herd of the United States was located. He said that the prize-winning herd for herds of 50 cows or over was located at Overbrook Hospital in New Jersey. I asked if he thought there was any chance of my being able to visit this herd. He thought it could be arranged, as he knew the dairyman in charge of the herd very well. In due time I received an invitation.

As production, feeding, and health of the herd were discussed during the visit I learned that a seaweed and fishmeal preparation was used as a ration supplement. He referred to it as *Manamar* and said that it was a form by which he could maintain more protein in the ration without risking sickness in his cows. This raised questions in my mind. Was it protein which represented the main problem in handling dairy herds? Did acid and potassium neutralize ill effects of protein, so that it was possible to get maximum milk production without injuring the health of the cow? This visit led naturally to study of protein-fed dairy cows.

Dairymen today have heard so much about protein that they must regard themselves as protein-conscious. When buying a bag of feed the first question is, "What is the percentage of protein?" Too often the questioning does not go beyond the percentage. A feed is 16, 18, 20, or 24 per cent protein, or whatever the percentage happens to be. The price tag and the anticipated results are largely estimated on the percentage of protein stated on the feed bag.

I will cite an example of the constructive value of combining acid with protein intake. The owner of a mixed herd of 54 dairy cows discussed with me his pet cow, a Jersey weighing 800 pounds. Two years earlier the bacteriologist at the local creamery and the local veterinary advised my farmer friend to get rid of this cow. But he happened to be particularly fond of her and kept postponing having her slaughtered for beef.

She had mastitis all the time. Each time her milk was checked by the local creamery bacteriologist, there would be streptococci present in the milk from each of the four quarters of her udder. It was finally decided that her usefulness had passed and that she should be disposed of.

She was due to give birth to her calf the early part of November. It was anticipated that the severity of the mastitis would increase when she freshened; the milk would increase with the birth of the calf, but it would be unfit to use.

I suggested to my friend that some of the trouble he was having might well be due to the fact that he was breaking a very old nutritional law pertaining to the seeds of plants. Whereas it required that acid be taken when the seeds of plants were used for food, this cow had not received sufficient roughage, such as acid leaves represent. Normally the cow should have been able to eat tender young leaves at the place on the plant where it showed its most recent growth.

It was immediately decided to pour one teaspoonful of apple cider vinegar per 100 pounds of the cow's body weight over her ration when it was placed in the trough. As she weighed 800 pounds, this meant adding 8 teaspoonfuls of the vinegar to the ration at each feeding. Since she got two feedings a day, she received 16 teaspoonfuls a day.

The day following the first addition of the vinegar, I telephoned my farmer friend to find out the cow's reaction. It seems that she had sniffed the ration a few times and then eaten it eagerly. When the ration was gone, she continued to lick the trough for half an hour. This proved that the apple cider vinegar represented something she wanted instinctively; hence it would be perfectly safe to continue it.

The vinegar was started two weeks before the birth of the calf, on

November 5. The cow's udder quieted down, the mastitis cleared up. After the birth all four quarters of the udder continued quiet, with no new development of mastitis. Sulfanilamide had previously been tried on this cow in an effort to control her mastitis. During the past two years, said my friend, he must have given the animal several pounds of sulfanilamide. It would seem to control the trouble for a little while, but then it would return.

After the cow was put on the apple cider vinegar it was possible to change the make-up of her ration and she began getting one half of a 16 per cent protein, and one half of a 14 per cent ration. On 9 pounds of grain, this little 800-pound Jersey cow was giving a 14-quart milk pail full (counting froth of about one inch) at each of the two milkings per day. This was about twice as good a record as the cow had made previously. And the apple cider vinegar got the credit for the improvement.

Her slaughter for beef was indefinitely postponed. By February 4 the quarters of her udder were perfect. She was eating well and feeding hearty. She was now giving 38 pounds of milk a day and getting 6 pounds of fitting ration, which is 14 per cent protein.

By May 1 she still continued normal, without any reappearance of mastitis. It was hard to decide who was the most interested in continuance of her apple cider vinegar allowance of 8 teaspoonfuls twice a day—she or her owner.

Following are conclusions arrived at from using apple cider vinegar in mastitis of the cow's udder:

1. Following disappearance of the mastitis, the original sponginess of the affected quarter will return. This sponginess is estimated by palpating the udder. This conclusion is based also on a return to normal of the amount of milk produced by this quarter.

2. Following the clearing up of the mastitis with the vinegar the quarter or quarters of the udder involved are smaller at first but at the end of two months will be filled out.

3. The small Jersey cow first treated with vinegar for chronic mastitis two years ago now has an udder that is as perfect as can be. This cow has become one of the best milk-producing members of the herd.

4. In an ordinary case of mastitis, a swollen quarter will return to normal size within one week after the apple cider vinegar is started. If an attack is severe, two months will be required to return such a quarter to its normal size.

5. As for salvaging cows that have chronic mastitis, about 75 per cent can be restored to profitability in the herd.

As a result of experimenting on this small Jersey cow, it was decided to try giving each cow in the herd two ounces of the vinegar, poured over the ration immediately it was placed in the feed trough, and see what happened. If it was the potassium which so greatly benefitted the first cow, then with confidence potassium could be added to the dairy farm soil, with the expectation of getting comparable results.

The first observation after the method went into operation was an increase in milk production by the herd. The following figures speak for themselves:

MILK PRODUCTION FIGURES OBTAINED FROM CREAMERY

	1943 52 Cows Without Vinegar	1944 54 Cows With Vinegar		1945 54 Cows With Vinegar
Jan. 1 to 15 ...	11,977 lbs.	17,662 lbs.		17,540 lbs.
Jan. 16 to 31 ..	13,542 "	17,716 "		17,662 "
Feb. 1 to 15 ...	14,190 "	16,243 "		16,516 "
Feb. 16 to 29 ..	12,899 "	14,204 "		14,170 "
Mar. 1 to 15 ...	15,354 "	14,846 "	Out of Vinegar	18,321 "
Mar. 16 to 31 ..	16,400 "	15,715 "		22,273 "
Apr. 1 to 15 ...	14,809 "	14,754 "	Vinegar Started	21,827 "
Apr. 16 to 30 ..	14,285 "	15,913 "		20,754 "
May 1 to 15 ...	15,754 "	18,819 "		18,665 "
May 16 to 31 ..	18,718 "	23,210 "		22,243 "
June 1 to 15 ...	18,328 "	21,863 "		19,854 "
June 16 to 30 ..	16,983 "	17,462 "		19,866 "
July 1 to 15 ...	16,580 "	15,265 "	No vinegar	18,285 "
July 16 to 31 ..	18,439 "	13,297 "		19,272 "
Aug. 1 to 15 ...	16,194 "	13,096 "		20,205 "
Aug. 16 to 31 ..	17,595 "	16,927 "	Vinegar Started	19,861 "
Sept. 1 to 15 ..	17,850 "	17,963 "		17,737 "
Sept. 16 to 30 ..	16,591 "	19,631 "		19,530 "
Oct. 1 to 15 ...	16,234 "	19,924 "		17,176 "
Oct. 16 to 31 ..	17,478 "	21,646 "		16,815 "
Nov. 1 to 15 ...	16,668 "	19,122 "		19,039 "
Nov. 16 to 30 ..	15,872 "	17,434 "		17,334 "
Dec. 1 to 15 ...	14,959 "	17,299 "		17,247 "
Dec. 16 to 31 ..	17,368 "	19,513 "		19,467 "

In the four weeks of March, 1944, this farmer was unable to obtain a supply of apple cider vinegar. This accounts for the drop in milk production shown by the figures. He then was able to obtain five barrels of vinegar. Milk production rose, but, as the figures show, it required two weeks to reach a milk increase over the previous year. During July and the first two weeks in August, 1944, the vinegar was not given because the herd was on pasture so it was thought unnecessary. But another drop in milk production made it clear that, since apple cider vinegar apparently contained elements lacking in the ration and pasture vegetation, it was as necessary during summer as winter months if herd milk production was to be maintained.

Let us consider the influence on the butterfat content of milk of two ounces of the vinegar poured over each cow's twice-a-day feeding.

This herd I was studying was a member of the Dairy Herd Improvement Association and was regularly checked by a cow tester employed by the association. This cow tester told me that of the 23 herds he tested regularly this Jersey registered herd had the highest milk butterfat content of them all. Addition of the apple cider vinegar to the ration was started November 1. During the month of the following April this herd tested 5.1 per cent butterfat. During the month of May this herd of 45 registered Jerseys had 27 quality cows. A quality cow is one that gives 1000 pounds of milk for a month with 40 pounds of butterfat. Twenty-seven was the greatest number of quality cows this herd had ever had; prior to this the greatest number at any one time was 19. During the following September the butterfat test of this herd was 5.61; this marked the highest butterfat test this herd had ever had.

The cow tester further told me that cows in all the other herds in the association were eating from 20 to 25 pounds of hay per cow per day, whereas the cows in this Jersey registered herd would only eat 13 pounds per day per cow when the vinegar was added to their ration. This lower consumption of hay represented a saving to the herd owner of $225.00 a month on hay alone. Charged against this was the cost of one barrel of vinegar per month, which was $18.00. The following figures are interesting evidence concerning the influence of apple cider vinegar on the amount of ration purchased for cows in a mixed herd:

January, February, and March 1944, 50 Cows in Mixed Herd
Amount paid for herd's ration at $42 a ton $1143.00
January, February, and March 1943, 52 Cows in Mixed Herd
Amount paid for herd's ration at $46 a ton $1212.00

January, February, and March 1944, 52 Cows in Mixed Herd

Two ounces of apple cider vinegar added to ration at each
    feeding

Amount paid for herd's ration at $65 a ton $1100.00

Without addition of the vinegar for these first three months in 1944,
based on the feed amounts purchased the first three months of 1942
and 1943, the 1944 3-month feed bill would have been $1755.00. By
inclusion of the vinegar with the ration, $655.00 was saved on the feed
bill. The vinegar bill for that period was $90.00.

The figures for consumption of ration in tons per cow are as follows:

January, February, March, 1942	0.54 tons per cow
January, February, March, 1943	0.51 tons per cow
January, February, March, 1944	0.31 tons per cow

My farmer friend reached the following conclusion from his experience with using the vinegar for his young stock. Given a choice between
two pounds of ration and no vinegar and a half pound of ration with
two ounces of vinegar added to it twice a day, he would choose the
latter because it would give his young stock the greatest growth in a
given period of time. I am well convinced that the potassium in the
vinegar is responsible for much of the good effect, since, as has often
been said in this book, potassium is associated with growth.

It seemed advisable to learn whether it was specifically the apple
cider vinegar that enabled the cow to balance increased protein intake,
or whether something associated with the acid was responsible for the
observed results.

It was noted that when a herd was turned for the first time into a
strip of pasture fertilized with acid phosphate, the cows would eat only
the grass on this strip, leaving the grass alone which grew on either side
of the strip. It was noted also that some cows would eat acid phosphate
if it was available. This led me to wonder whether if phosphoric acid
were poured over the ration of a few cows the same results would be
produced as by adding the apple cider vinegar to the ration of other
cows in the herd.

Five cows were selected for this experiment. They were taken off the
vinegar supplement and put on a phosphoric acid supplement of one
teaspoonful of the acid poured over the ration twice each day.

Nothing happened until nearly two weeks had passed. Then one or
more quarters of each cow's udder began to swell. The phosphoric acid
was immediately discontinued and the vinegar restored, whereupon the
swollen quarters returned to normal.

APPENDIX B

SOME OTHER USES OF APPLE CIDER VINEGAR IN VERMONT FOLK MEDICINE

Liniment to Relieve Lameness

Beat up yolk of one egg with one tablespoonful of turpentine and one tablespoonful of apple cider vinegar. Apply this to the skin surface, rubbing well in, to relieve lameness.

Poison Ivy

Use equal parts of apple cider vinegar and water. Dab on the affected part and allow to dry on the skin. Apply often.

Shingles

Apply apple cider vinegar, just as it comes from the bottle, to the skin area where the shingles are located, four times during the day and three times during the night if you are awake. The itching and burning sensation in the skin will leave in a few minutes after the vinegar is applied, and the shingles will heal more readily with this treatment.

Night Sweats

If the skin surface of the body is given a cupped-palm hand bath of apple cider vinegar at bedtime, the night sweats will be prevented.

Burns

Undiluted apple cider vinegar, just as it comes from the bottle, if applied to a burn on the surface of the body, will remove all smarting and soreness.

To Shrink Varicose Veins

This is not only a remedy of Vermont folk medicine but, I learn from patients, is also a remedy of folk medicine in Scotland, England,

173

and Germany. Apply apple cider vinegar, just as it comes from the bottle, to the varicose veins night and morning, by means of the cupped-hands treatment. Shrinking of the veins will be noticed at the end of the month. In addition to applying the vinegar to the veins, two tea-spoonfuls of vinegar in a glass of water are taken twice a day.

Impetigo

Undoubtedly, impetigo is the "catchingest" disease in the world. It may be caught from one touch of a finger or one dab of a towel. Usually it begins as a red or pimply spot no bigger than a split pea. Often it appears on the cheek or around the nose, where it may be mistaken for a cold sore. Soon it begins to enlarge, blister, discharge, and spread to other parts of the body. Finally the blistery eruption dries into a yellow crust that is loosely attached.

Technically, impetigo is a staphylococcus or streptococcus infection of the skin. Anybody of any age may catch it, but children seem to be especially susceptible. Indeed, unless a patient strictly keeps his hands off his sores, he may have crop after crop, indefinitely. If, however, he controls himself, he may be well and presentable in two weeks.

In treating impetigo, use apple cider vinegar just as it comes from the bottle. Dip the finger in it and apply to each affected part of the skin. Application should be six times a day, beginning on rising in the morning and at intervals to bedtime. As a rule the impetigo will have disappeared in two to four days.

Ringworm

For some years ringworm of the scalp has been spreading over the United States. Most commonly, the ringworm areas are rounded, scaly patches, small in size, which appear at first glance to be bald patches. Close inspection, however, will reveal hair shafts broken off close to the scalp. The ringworm patches may or may not show local inflammation. When inflammation is present, it may vary from a mild low-grade inflammation, with usually a few crusts present, through all the stages up to a marked redness, with some swelling of tissue and pus points. Glands not far from the ringworm may be enlarged. The patches of ringworm may be single or multiple. They are most frequent on or above the back of the head, but they can appear wherever the hair is growing. Though spontaneous cures are sometimes seen, the majority of lesions tend to persist indefinitely if left untreated.

Boys are affected six to nine times more often than girls. Ringworm is due to a fungus which is transmitted directly from child to child. It may also be transmitted to children from cats and dogs. The spread of ringworm seems to be largely by way of swapped hats and caps or high-backed seats in theaters and conveyances, where children's heads can rub against the upholstery.

Apply apple cider vinegar with the fingers to the ringworm area six times a day, beginning on rising in the morning and continuing through to bedtime. Apple cider vinegar is an excellent antiseptic.

APPENDIX C

VERMONT FOLK MEDICINE AND BEVERAGES

Treatment for Hangover

During the passing years, Vermont folk medicine has learned by the trial and error method how to deal successfully with sobering up the individual who has been on a drinking spree. A man in his forties had been drinking from December 27 to January 10. He was paralyzed drunk when seen. He was given six teaspoonfuls of honey. Twenty minutes later he was given another six teaspoonfuls, and twenty minutes later a third dose in the same amount. This made 18 teaspoonfuls of honey in 40 minutes. Beside his bed was a fifth of liquor, with one drink left in the bottle. Three hours later the drink was still there. Treatment was continued: three doses of six teaspoonfuls of honey each, repeated at 20-minute intervals.

The following morning he was seen at 8:30. He had slept straight through the night until 7:30 A.M. This was something he had not experienced for 20 years. He had, however, taken the one remaining drink of liquor. First he was given three more doses of six teaspoonfuls of honey at intervals of 20 minutes. He was then given a soft-boiled egg. Ten minutes later he received six teaspoonfuls of honey. His lunch consisted of four teaspoonfuls of honey at the beginning of the meal, a glass of tomato juice, and a piece of ground beef. For dessert he received four more teaspoonfuls of honey.

A friend brought him a pint of liquor, which was placed on the table with his evening meal. He pushed it away, and said he did not want it any more. He never took another drink again.

As a result of the honey given this man, a paralyzed drunk at 7:00 P.M. was made sober within 24 hours with the help of 2 pounds of honey. Vermont folk medicine considers overindulgence in alcohol to

176

be evidence of potassium deficiency in the body. Being a good source of potassium, honey counteracts the craving for alcohol and successfully accomplishes the sobering-up process.

In this connection I undertook to learn the reaction of alcoholic beverages when tested with Squibb's Nitrazine Paper. With the cooperation of a bartender friend who brought samples to my office of the different alcoholic beverages sold over the bar, I tested them with the different waters used in mixing drinks. Their reactions lined up as follows:

Beverage	*Reaction*
Whisky	pH 6.0 weakly acid
Rum	pH 5.5 acid
Vichy Water	pH 7.0 weakly alkaline
Beer	pH 4.5 very acid
Sparkling Water	pH 5.5 acid
Sherry Wine	pH 4.5 very acid
Port Wine	pH 4.5 " "
Vermouth	pH 4.5 " "
Creme de Menthe	pH 6.0 weakly acid
Gin	pH 6.0 " "

If we remember the instinct in dairy cows and human beings which causes them to seek an acid, we can better understand why the laborer enjoys a bottle of beer, with its very acid pH of 4.5, at the end of a hard day's work. We can better understand why the business and professional man often enjoys a cocktail before the evening meal. The alcoholic beverage, which is acid in reaction, satisfies the instinctive desire for an acid. It is interesting to note that wines and beer are the most acid of all alcoholic beverages.

The fact that coffee and tea are both extremely acid beverages, having a reaction of pH 4.5, makes it easy to understand their popularity as beverages. In Vermont folk medicine often the only liquid taken when sickness appears is tea.

I also tested soda-fountain beverages, and beverages sold in grocery stores in Barre. I learned their reactions as follows, using the Squibb's Nitrazine Paper:

REACTION OF SODA FOUNTAIN BEVERAGES

Beverage	*Reaction*
Coca Cola	pH 4.5 very acid
Hire's Root Beer	pH 6.0 acid
Moxie	pH 4.5 very acid
Yukon Club Pale Dry Ginger Ale	pH 4.5 " "
Lemon and Lime	pH 4.5 " "
Pepsi Cola	pH 4.5 " "
Orange Crush	pH 4.5 " "

REACTION OF BEVERAGES SOLD AT GROCERY STORES

Beverage	*Reaction*
Vegetable Juice Cocktail	pH 4.5 very acid
Carrot Juice	" " "
Apricot Juice	" " "
Cranberry Juice	" " "
Prune Juice	" " "
Grape Juice	" " "
Orange Juice	" " "
Apple Juice	" " "
Tea	" " "
Coffee	" " "

With the exception of Hire's Root Beer all the above beverages are extremely acid, being pH 4.5. Hire's Root Beer is weakly acid. The volume purchase at drugstores of these acid beverages indicates the instinctive craving of the body for an acid.

APPENDIX D

CHEMICAL ANALYSIS OF KELP

I went to spend a day at Cornell University with the late George W. Cavanaugh, Professor of Agricultural Chemistry. Ocean kelp was his research hobby, and we had several discussions about it. It was his opinion that the human body greatly needed a food supplement to meet the exacting requirements of our present environment and life tempo.

He first presented the following analysis of sea kelp: *

Moisture	6.00%
Protein (crude)	7.50%
Fiber (crude)	7.20%
Nitrogen (free extract)	45.28%
Fat (ether extract)	0.34%
Ash	33.68%
	100.00%

APPROXIMATE COMPOSITION OF ASH

Mineral Elements	Per Cent
Calcium	1.00
Phosphorus	.34
Magnesium	.74
Sodium	4.00
Potassium	12.00
Clorine	13.37
Sulfur	1.00
Iron	.04
Iodine	.19
Undetermined	1.00
Total	33.68%

* I am indebted to the late George W. Cavanaugh, Professor of Agricultural Chemistry at Cornell University, for the following two tables.

In the spectrographic analysis of kelp *(Macrocystic pyrifera)* issued by the United States Bureau of Fisheries, the elements recognized by definite light are given in the following table.

SPECTROGRAPHIC QUALITATIVE ANALYSIS OF SAMPLE OF ASH FROM KELP

Element	Estimated Quantity
Sodium	over 10.0%
Potassium	over 10.0%
Calcium	over 10.0%
Iron	0.1%
Aluminum	0.1%
Magnesium	0.1%
Strontium	0.1%
Silicon	0.01 to 0.1%
Manganese	0.01 to 0.1%
Copper	0.001 to 0.01%
Tin	0.001 to 0.01%
Lead	0.001 to 0.01%
Vanadium	0.001%
Zinc	0.001%
Titanium	0.0001 to 0.001%
Chromium	0.0001 to 0.001%
Barium	0.0001 to 0.001%
Silver	0.0001%

As for vitamin content, kelp is an excellent source of vitamin A and vitamin E. It is a good source of vitamin B and contains vitamin D.

Unpublished data by Professor Cavanaugh at the time of my visit showed that kelp contains generous amounts of mannitol, a gentle purgative and bile stimulant; small amounts of lecithin, a phosphorus compound thought to be of great importance in the knitting of broken bones, especially in old people; and carotin, the parent substance of vitamin A.

EACH TEASPOONFUL OF KELP CONTAINS THE FOLLOWING

1/10 grain organic iodine
3/5 grain organic calcium
7 grains organic potassium
½ grain organic sulfur
½ grain organic magnesium

1/45 grain organic iron
1/1800 grain organic copper
1/6 grain organic phosphorus
2½ grains organic sodium

APPENDIX E

HARMFUL BACTERIA AND ALKALINITY

A friend on the faculty of a medical school sent me for my information a list of bacteria harmful to the human body, with the reaction of the media most favorable for their growth. This list was made up for me at his request by the department of bacteriology, and reads as follows:

MOST FAVORABLE REACTION OF MEDIA FOR GROWING PATHOGENIC BACTERIA

Microorganism	Reaction	
Staphylococcus	7.4	alkaline
Streptococcus	7.4 to 7.6	"
Pneumococcus	7.6 to 7.8	"
H. Influenza	7.8	"
Meningococcus	7.4 to 7.6	"
Gonococcus	7.0 to 7.4	"
Corymbacterium diptheriae	7.2	"
B. abortus	7.2 to 7.4	"
B. tularemae	6.8 to 7.3	"
Clostridium tetani	7.0 to 7.6	"

It becomes apparent, as one studies this list, that microorganisms harmful to the human body grow on an alkaline soil. This is particularly interesting in the light of the evidence that in dairy cows and human beings alike, an instinct exists which leads them to seek an acid intake.

In the light of the above evidence, it seems reasonable to suspect that pathogenic bacteria which are harmful to the body are in the world for another purpose than to cause sickness in human beings. Nature has spread acid vegetation about with a lavish hand, apparently to prevent infestation of the body with pathogenic microorganisms, turning into infection of the body by these same microorganisms. The instinct leading animals and humans to seek acid vegetation and acid liquids has been given as a protection.